RENEWALS 458-4574

DATE DUE

DEC 2 6			
DEC - 6			
APR 1 9			
MAY 1 8 2000			
MAY 1 3			
NOV 1 1			
MAY 1 9			
OCT 2 8 2008			
NOV 2 6 2008			
FEB 2 6 2009			
MAR 2 6 2009			
GAYLORD			PRINTED IN U.S.A.

EPIDEMIC IN THE SOUTHWEST
1918 - 1919

SOUTHWESTERN STUDIES

MONOGRAPH NO. 72

Epidemic in the Southwest
1918 - 1919

by

Bradford Luckingham

COPYRIGHT 1984
TEXAS WESTERN PRESS
The University of Texas at El Paso

ISBN 0-87404-148-1

ABOUT THE AUTHOR

Bradford Luckingham, member of the History Department faculty at Arizona State University, Tempe, since 1971, is a specialist in urban history of the American West. His book, *"The Urban Southwest, A Profile History of Albuquerque, El Paso, Phoenix and Tucson,"* was published by Texas Western Press in 1982. Currently he is working on a comprehensive history of the city of Phoenix. His long range plans include a work of considerable scope, dealing with the role of the city in the growth and development of the American West.

The author holds a B.A. degree from Northern Arizona University in Flagstaff; an M.A. degree from the University of Missouri, Columbia; and a Ph.D. from the University of California at Davis. He is a member of the Western History Association and the Arizona Historical Society. Luckingham has published articles in numerous journals, among them the *Missouri Historical Review, Mid-America, Journal of Negro History, Southern California Quarterly, Journal of the West, Journal of Arizona History, Western Historical Quarterly,* and the *Journal of Urban History.*

"Spanish" Influenza—"The Flu"
"Three-Day Fever"

The disease now spreading over this country is highly catching and may invade your community and attack you and your family unless you are very careful.

INFLUENZA is a crowd disease. *Therefore:* **Keep out of crowds as much as possible.**

INFLUENZA probably spreads mostly by inhaling some of the tiny droplets of germ-laden mucus sprayed into the air when ignorant or careless persons sneeze or cough without using a handkerchief. *Therefore:* **Cover up each cough and sneeze.**

INFLUENZA is probably spread also by the filthy habit of spitting on sidewalks, street cars, and other public places. *Therefore:* **Do not spit on the floor or sidewalk.**

INFLUENZA is probably spread also by the use of common drinking cups and the use of common towels in public places. *Therefore:* **Shun the common drinking cup and the roller towel in public places.**

If you feel sick and believe you have "Spanish" Influenza, go to bed and send for the doctor. This is important.

All that has been said above about "Spanish" Influenza is true also of Colds, Bronchitis, Pneumonia, and Tuberculosis. Do your part to keep them away.

RUPERT BLUE,
Surgeon General,
U. S. Public Health Service.

Above is one of the numerous health notices distributed to cities throughout the nation by the Surgeon General, U.S. Public Health Service, during the devastating influenza epidemic of 1918-1919.

COURTESY THE J.H. McCLINTOCK COLLECTION, PHOENIX PUBLIC LIBRARY

EPIDEMIC IN THE SOUTHWEST
1918 - 1919

Chapter I
A NATIONAL DISASTER

In October 1918, the front pages of the nation's newspapers were filled with news of World War I. Headlines depicted the steady advance of Allied troops in Europe, as Americans helped crush German resistance in battle after battle. Each day, reports from the front declared that victory was near at hand.

While Americans eagerly awaited the end of the war in Europe, they were also combating the ravages of a devastating influenza epidemic at home. In Europe the disease had been labeled the Spanish influenza, and from that beleaguered continent the germ had spread to every part of the world. In a short period of time, twenty million people succumbed to the dread disease. The *London Times* stated that "never since the Black Death has such a plague swept the world." It was a global calamity that invaded the east coast of the United States and quickly moved westward across the country with deadly effect. By the time peace negotiations in Europe commenced in November 1918, every state in the U.S. had been invaded by the epidemic. In fact, more than ten times as many Americans were killed by the disease as were killed by German bombs and bullets during World War I.[1]

In the nation's cities, the disease struck quickly. In one week in October, 4,500 died in Philadelphia, and 3,200 died in Chicago. "In most cases," declared Surgeon General Rupert Blue of the United States

Public Health Service, "a person taken sick with Spanish influenza feels sick rather suddenly. He feels weak, has pains in the eyes, ears, head or back, abdomen, etc., and may be sore all over." He continued: "Ordinarily the fever lasts from three to four days and the patient recovers. But while the proportion of deaths is usually low, in some places the outbreak is severe and deaths are numerous. When death occurs, it is usually the result of the development of pneumonia or of some other complication." Surgeon General Blue and his staff sent out reams of advice to community officials, but nothing seemed to work. Medical knowledge had expanded in recent years, but influenza yielded to no known medication or technique. Dr. Blue and other medical men had to rely on the most rudimentary public and personal health measures.[2]

As the epidemic spread, health offiicials in many cities closed meeting places such as schools, churches, and theatres, and prohibited all public gatherings. New ordinances appeared that made it a crime to cough or sneeze or spit in public, and which required individuals to wear face masks in public. Physicians prescribed every conceivable remedy, including alcohol consumption; they also warned against kissing and shaking hands. All kinds of vaccines were tried. But the epidemic continued to rage in America's urban centers. Hospitals and cemeteries were filled to capacity. On October 10, 1918, in Philadelphia, 759 victims of Spanish influenza and its complications died. Bodies piled up in the city morgue where conditions became "so offensive that veteran embalmers recoiled and refused to enter." A coffin shortage forced some city governments to manufacture them. A Buffalo, New York, health official noted that "they will not be $1,000 or even $100 caskets," but "plain caskets."[3]

Public and private services lagged behind. Police and fire forces were reduced by the disease. Sanitation workers and streetcar conductors, office clerks and telephone operators, caught the "flu bug." The *New York Times* urged its readers to make no unnecessary phone calls because 2,000 of the city's telephone operators had influenza. Factories closed. Weddings were postponed. Conventions were cancelled. Entire families were wiped out. Doctors and nurses who escaped the contagion were vastly overworked.[4]

Countless volunteers, ranging from society matrons to social workers, responded to the increasing demands for help. Despite the odds, the "Battle of the Flu" was fought unceasingly in city after city. Along with food, clothing, and care for the victims, many citizens contributed in other ways in the attempts to prevent the epidemic from spreading further. People turned their homes into soup kitchens, their automobiles into ambulances, and their schools, churches, and clubs into emergency hospitals. Examples of genuine concern were evident in every city in America, and those countless individuals who volunteered their services earned the satisfaction of lending a helping hand to less fortunate fellow citizens in their hour of need. And many of them lost their lives in the effort.

Urban women everywhere in the nation comprised the majority of the volunteers. In Philadelphia, for example, "they acted as nurses, staffed the soup kitchens, answered the phones, cooked and cleaned for the helpless, sewed shrouds, calmed the frantic and comforted the bereaved, drove the ambulances, and closed the eyes of the dead." Time and again observers declared that the individual and collective efforts of volunteers were a great contribution in coping with the explosion of community crises in urban America. Indeed, a Harvard professor, writing of Boston's influenza epidemic, expressed admiration for the ability of that city's community-minded citizens to "organize themselves for an emergency." During the epidemic they not only tried to make "the city of Boston a safer place to live in, but also a place in which one may be proud to live."⁵

Nobody knew where the Spanish influenza came from, or how it was communicated. The very mystery of the disease bred fear. Observers even asserted that the influenza germs had been brought to America by German agents put ashore from submarines at unguarded locations along the Atlantic coast. Critics of the germ warfare theory, however, noted that thousands of Germans in Europe were also dying from the disease. The same pattern existed everywhere. There appeared to be no escape from the grip of Spanish influenza. Evangelist Billy Sunday thought he had the answer; as he put it to a New York City audience in October: "We can pray down an epidemic just as well as we can pray down a German victory." At the same time, 800 people a day were dying in New York City from the disease and its complications. Before the epidemic ended in that urban center, 19,000 died. In Boston, children were heard singing a new song:

> I had a little bird
> And its name was Enza.
> I opened the window
> And in - flew - Enza.⁶

With a patient in every bed in every hospital in Washington, D.C., the national capitol found itself in a critical situation. The Senate and

the House of Representatives closed their galleries to everyone except
reporters, and the Supreme Court adjourned to avoid bringing lawyers
to what Justice Oliver Wendell Holmes called "this crowded and infected place." Every office of every department of the federal government was only partially staffed, due to the absence of employees who
had contracted the flu. To make room for new admissions to
Washington hospitals, undertakers were stationed at the doors, ready
to remove bodies as fast as the victims died. "The living come in one
door and the dead went out the other," lamented a doctor. Some local
undertakers, called "the coffin trust" by critics, took advantage of the
crisis by overcharging grieving families for funerals. Profiteering was
rampant, in fact, the mayor of New York City heard so many complaints about overcharging by doctors and druggists that he threatened
to have their names published in the press. At the same time, honest
and conscientious business interests complained of the rules and regulations imposed upon them because of the epidemic. Theatre owners, for
example, wondered why they should be forced to close and make financial sacrifices, while local officials left others, engaged in certain enter-
tainment enterprises, to remain open for business.[7]

The war effort of course continued throughout the epidemic. At
home, in spite of the many health rules and regulations, liberty bond
drives and draft calls proceeded on schedule. Headlines, signifying
Allied victories over the Germans, bannered the front pages of the nation's newspapers. On November 11, 1918, many of the nation's urban
dwellers turned out to celebrate the armistice and the coming of peace
in Europe. "Multitudes poured forth," stated the *Philadelphia In-
quirer*, "from the stately mansions of the rich, from the modest homes
and lodgings of the workers, from the alleys and the courts of the lowly
and the poor." Fortunately, by that time the Spanish influenza
epidemic had begun to dissipate as inexplicably as it had begun. The
number of new cases and deaths declined rapidly in many of the nation's cities, but some in both the East and the West were to experience
a second wave of the dread disease.[8]

The Spanish influenza moved from East to West in much the same
direction as the pioneers had moved westward, and although the
disease tended to arrive later and end later in the cities of the West, it
was just as devastating to its victims. In Denver and Seattle, Los
Angeles and San Francisco, local officials tried every technique, procedure, and remedy that had been used in the eastern cities in the effort
to cure or slow the advance of the deadly malady. All types of informa-

tion, on how to avoid or survive influenza, was disseminated to the public and the press. Public gatherings were prohibited. All schools, churches, and places of public amusement such as theatres, were closed. Many citizens were inoculated with useless vaccines. In San Francisco and other western cities, health officials also spent much time and effort trying to persuade people to wear anti-influenza germ masks. Yet, despite widespread utilization in the urban Far West of all known preventatives and treatments for influenza, and despite the enforcement of various rules and regulations for the control of the disease as stringent as any implemented in any of the cities of the East, the cities of the West did not escape the full force of the epidemic. In San Francisco, for example, there were over 50,000 reported cases of Spanish influenza, and 3,500 of them died from the disease and its complications.[9]

The urban centers of the Southwest also fought the Battle of the Flu. Each of the major cities of that region, El Paso, Albuquerque, Tucson, and Phoenix, faced a community crisis in the fall of 1918. The detailed story of how each of them responded to the Spanish influenza epidemic is told in the following chapters.[10]

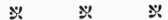

Chapter II

EL PASO
A Community Crisi

El Paso, Texas, with a population approac... 75,000 in September 1918, was the largest city in the Southwest. A railroad hub and an industrial center, it served a vast hinterland of mining, farming, and cattle interests. The border city, located across the Rio Grande River from Juarez, Mexico, also was a health haven and tourist attraction. In addition, the city served as the home of Fort Bliss, the leading military installation in the region. First the Mexican Revolution and then World War I contributed to the rapid development of Fort Bliss. During the revolt, troops from the El Paso post were employed to protect the border, and during the European conflict the post played an important role as a training center for thousands of soldiers. Unfortunately, during the fall of 1918 Fort Bliss and many other army posts around the country could not avoid the "clutch of Spanish influenza."[1]

On September 25, the *El Paso Times* noted the presence of the disease in 25 army camps, including some in Texas, but not at Fort Bliss. "There is no cause for alarm in El Paso," the paper asserted, but "it is well to acquaint ourselves with something we may have to contend with later." By October 3, less than two weeks later, El Paso had 250 cases of Spanish influenza, with most of those at Fort Bliss. The post was placed under quarantine. City officials forbade the gathering of crowds and ordered the closing of all schools, churches, theatres, and other public meeting places in El Paso. Police Chief Charles Pollock received instructions from Mayor Charles Davis to enforce the orders.

Dr. Hugh White, city health officer, cautioned the public not to be alarmed, but to be on the alert. "There is no reason to get panicky over the present situation in the city," stated Dr. John W. Tappan, medical officer in charge of the United States Public Health Service in El Paso, "yet at the rate the disease is increasing, every rule for its control should be observed." He went on to say that "since quarantine in this disease is impracticable, too much stress cannot be placed upon the avoidance of crowds, and closing places helps." All "measures which are recognized by the federal government as prophylactic should be enforced in El Paso. Better an ounce of prevention than a pound of cure."[2]

On October 8, El Paso officials estimated 1,800 Spanish influenza cases in the city, about half of them at Fort Bliss. Post and city hospitals were filled to capacity, and the call was out for more doctors and nurses. "Nurses are almost impossible to get and doctors are scarce and overworked," a hospital spokesman lamented. He deplored the "present rate of increase" in influenza cases and pleaded with the public "to observe every precautionary measure that is possible." Red Cross workers helped by furnishing 1,500 masks for nurses and doctors who were fighting the flu. Volunteers offered their services day and night. Emergency training courses taught "home care of the sick." Undertakers could not keep up with the increasing need for their services. City officials issued more orders: no overcrowding of streetcars; no funerals conducted in churches; no dances. All physicians in the city were told to report all new cases of influenza to the health department at city hall as soon as possible. And before long, Juarez, Mexico, (just across the river) was as hard hit as El Paso.[3]

Mexican-Americans living in south El Paso quickly presented the most serious problem. On October 15, the *Times* announced 37 deaths from influenza in that section of the city. The epidemic in south El Paso multiplied the work of the Associated Charities, and members of that organization stated that conditions "south of the tracks" were deplorable. Mrs. C.B. Hooper found 22 sick people in one house. Public and private agencies offered free care and free burials, and city officials ordered a "clean up" of south El Paso. "Sanitary commissioner L.D. Hullum is taking no chances on the south side and has 16 wagons working continuously gathering garbage, hoping in this way to combat the spread of influenza," declared the *El Paso Herald*. Hullum reported "the south side cleaner than it has been for many years."[4]

The troops at Fort Bliss, where there were 2,000 cases on October 15, remained under strict quarantine. Any soldiers found on the streets of El Paso without permission were arrested. Morever, those who were given "special permission" to enter the city were forbidden to go south of Overland Street, one of the main thoroughfares downtown. In this respect, the epidemic contributed to the steady decline of Anglo-Mexican relations in El Paso. A few Mexicans in the city enjoyed wealth and status, but most of them lived on the south side in a section known as "Chihuahuita" because so many immigrants from the Mexican state of Chihuahua had settled there. Poverty and destitution marked the area, and few Anglos settled there. Floods occasionally ravaged this lower part of town by the Rio Grande, and municipal utility services did not extend to many parts of that area. For example, while a paving program was proceeding elsewhere in the city, south El Paso streets remained alternately dusty and muddy in dry and wet weather. Although El Paso's rapid population growth was due in part to the ongoing migration from across the border, the Mexicans who resided in the city realized few of the benefits derived from local development. By 1918, the majority of the Mexicans employed in El Paso held low-level jobs, yet for many of them it seemed indeed better than being in Mexico's interior or its northern-most city, Juarez, where even less economic opportunity was available.[5]

Moreover, since 1910 the Mexican Revolution had brought great turmoil and devastation to northern Mexico and Juarez, and this caused a massive migration of Mexicans to El Paso. Although the refugees represented all economic levels, with the city profiting especially from the presence of the affluent, most of the newcomers were poor and as they settled in "Chihuahuita" they contributed to the problems already evident in that community. The *Herald* described the area as "a slum," and indicated that improvement of the Mexican quarters in El Paso was long overdue: "The city has not only neglected the elementary welfare of half its population, but it has tolerated conditions in that section that have constituted a terrible menace to all the rest of the city."

For the most part, however, Anglo El Paso ignored the deplorable conditions in the Mexican community "south of the tracks." In turn, the Mexicans in the barrios offered little resistance to discrimination and segregation, and so accommodation became the norm. Political apathy and corruption existed, and fear of Anglo reprisals to Mexican protests did not help the situation. Efforts to "Americanize" the Mexicans were thwarted, since many of them considered themselves only temporary stateside residents and wanted to retain their Mexican cultural identity. Since they hoped to return to Mexico as soon as they acquired sufficient means, they felt little or no loyalty to "Chihuahuita" or to El

Paso. Also, many Mexicans continued to consider the conditions in the south side neighborhoods superior to those in Juarez, or, for that matter, anywhere else in Mexico.[6]

As the decade evolved, problems in Mexican El Paso mounted. General John J. Pershing, commander of Fort Bliss, became so concerned about the effect the unsanitary environment in south El Paso was having on his troops that he volunteered the services of his medical officers to help the city clean up the place. Pershing also urged a health survey of the area, and a report was completed in September 1916. According to the director of the survey, El Paso's "first big problem is the Mexican condition and the unsanitary tenement houses that abound throughout the southern end of the city." The report noted that "probably in no place in the United States could such crude, beastly, primitive conditions be found as exist in 'Chihuahuita.' The condition of this section is largely an economic one and the treatment should be radical."[7]

The epidemic took its toll in south El Paso. The area lacked hospitals and other health services. Mexicans died from the lack of physicians, nurses, and care. Finally, plans for the hospitalization of Mexican sufferers of the disease were worked out by the city council, city board of health, city school board, the United States Public Health Service, the Red Cross, and the Associated Charities. It was decided on October 16 to convert the 28-room Aoy School into an emergency hospital "for influenza patients in the lower part of the city." The plan was to be "entirely cooperative" with the city furnishing the utilities; the school board providing the building; the United States Public Health Service supplying the physicians; the Red Cross contributing beds, medicines, nurses; and the Associated Charities taking care of the dependents of hospital patients. Located at Seventh Avenue and Kansas Street deep in south El Paso, the "new hospital" helped solve the problem of a scarcity of graduate nurses, the *Herald* stated, because "a few expert nurses, assisted by nongraduate nurses, could care for large numbers of patients." A "hygenic and sanitary" place was certainly needed by the time it opened on October 18, for the board of health reported 131 deaths from influenza in El Paso during the previous week, 102 of them Mexicans.[8]

The Aoy School emergency hospital proved to be a important aspect of El Paso's response to community crisis. People from all sections of the city volunteered their services. They prepared food and donated clothing. They used their automobiles as ambulances. El Paso women of all ages worked as cooks, clerks, drivers, and nurses aides. As one determined lady put it, "I am so glad to find that I can help. I have not had a nurses aide course, nor, in fact, any training. I probably have no qualifications for nursing except my desire to relieve some of the suffering." And Aoy School emergency hospital was filled with patients. "Fifty-one Mexican men, women and babies lay gasping in the improvised wards of Aoy School last night," wrote R.J. Pritchard of the *Times* on October 19. Brought in from "the squalor of homes in the Mexican quarter of town, many of them in the last stages of pneumonia, all of them suffering from the lack of proper medical attention and comforts, the patients were transferred from the depths of poverty to the comparative comfort and care of a hospital equal in almost every respect to any in the city."

Pritchard noted how individuals and organizations in the public and private sectors of El Paso had combined to create, within a short time, an emergency hospital with facilities for 100 patients. In the hospital, he saw "Mexicans of every age, and in every stage of the disease," and he described how they "lay tossing on canvas army cots in the throes of acute pneumonia, or else lay still, with faces upturned to the ceiling, eyes glassy, and only their heaving chests and whistling breath portraying the extent of their agony." In one ward "lay a grizzled Mexican," Pritchard continued, "tossing from side to side, his body in constant motion as he groaned perpetually for breath. Beside him on the next cot lay a small baby, hardly more than two months old, its brown hands clenched on the coverlet and its tiny black head motionless upon the pillow." Across the ward "an old woman sat on the edge of a cot, on which lay a child about 10 years old. Of the two the old woman was by far the most pitiful as she bent her aged head over the dying body of perhaps her youngest son." On another cot, a "young mother, not more than 18 years old, sat upright, clasping in her arms with a convulsive grip a three-month-old child. Careless of her own exposure, which might mean her death, the maternal spirit dominated her being to the exclusion of all else, as she fondled her cough-racked baby."[9]

Dr. W. L. Brown, assisted by an able corps of trained nurses and volunteers, served as head of the hospital, while Miss Katherine Gorbutt, principal of Aoy School, acted as custodian and general business manager of the institution. Sanitary conditions, according to observers, were remarkable considering the speed with which the emergency hospital was established. The "domestic science rooms have been converted into a kitchen, where beef broth and nourishing vegetable soups and other dietary nutriment is prepared," stated the *Times,* while "sufficient tin cups, plates and other utensils have been provided to take care of every patient, and every dish is thoroughly boiled after every meal." White garbed doctors, nurses, and attendants did their best to alleviate the situation, but the hospital was understaffed. Miss A. Louise Dietrich began training local women for duty in the El Paso Nurses' Aide Corps, and many of them served at the emergency hospital.

On October 19, Robert Krakauer, president of the Associated Charities, announced that the organization "urgently needs a fund of money for the relief of wives and children of wage earners on the south side who are down and out with influenza and pneumonia, many of them dying." He noted that the "Red Cross is doing wonderful work for the sick in Aoy hospital and are searching through the southside for those who should have medical treatment and nursing," but it is "not doing the family relief work, providing the hungry ones with food and clothing, because it is distinctly the charity associations business to do that, while the Red Cross takes the ones who must have medicine and care." While "the Red Cross workers are doing their best," Krakauer declared, "let us try to save the families who are not in bed, but hungry and cold."[10]

El Pasoans responded to the medical crisis in their community in an impressive way. Many Anglos and Mexicans, despite the hazards to their health, joined in the effort to stem the epidemic. It was crucial to secure Spanish-speaking volunteers to work the south side barrios, for many influenza victims in those neighborhoods refused or proved reluctant to go to the Aoy School emergency hospital. They did not want to leave home, family, and folk medicine to stay at a strange place and be treated by strange people; "They fear the hospital," noted an observer. Thus, Spanish-speaking volunteers capable of communicating with victims of the disease, played an important role in convincing the flu victims that the hospital and its services were working to alleviate their suffering. At the same time, according to city health inspector L.T. Jones, there remained many more Mexicans on the south side suffering from influenza than the reports indicated. "While many of the Mexican residents show a willingness to be taken to the hospital," Jones asserted, "numbers of others, reported to be ill, refuse to accompany the inspectors to the hospital, and remain ill in their homes."

Members of the Mexican community donated not only their time and skills, but also money and materials. Appeals in the Spanish language were prepared by Red Cross workers for the "special attention of the higher class of Mexicans in the city," telling them of the great need for volunteer help in south El Paso. Officers of the Casino Mexicano, a new social club composed of prominent Mexican businessmen in El Paso, solicited contributions from Mexican residents to aid influenza sufferers in the "southern part of the city." Mexican businesses donated products; for example, La Victoria bakery provided bread. At the emergency hospital, family members, friends, and others directly involved with the grim statistics expressed deep concern. The *Times* observed that "priests come daily to visit the sick, refusing to wear the protection masks as some of the patients cannot hear them, but can see their lips move."[11]

While many volunteers worked at the Aoy School emergency hospital, others helped out at Rolston, Providence, Hotel Dieu, and the post hospital at Fort Bliss. Since all of El Paso's hospitals were extremely busy during the crisis, they appreciated the services of volunteers. On October 23, for instance, Sister Demetria and her Hotel Dieu colleagues offered "a tribute of gratitude to all who assisted by word or deed during the past weeks of care and anxiety attendant on the prevailing epidemic affecting our city and people." Dr. Tappan of the United States Public Health Service also praised the "wonderful work" being done at the hospitals, and he believed that the Red Cross and other organizations cooperating at the Aoy School deserved "special credit." At the same time, Mrs. Clifford Hall, night supervisor at the institution, suggested that more could be done if more residents of south El Paso would cooperate. "There is room for more patients in the hospital and it is hoped that every place will be filled by those who need our attention," Hall declared. It "is a pity that we have places here, and so many Mexicans should remain at their home and suffer for the bare necessities of life. It is hoped that all who know of Mexicans needing attention and medical care will report them to the hospital so that they may be given treatment."

She also noted that there existed "much destitution among the Mexicans, and the hospital is without funds to aid in its outside work." There "is not much benefit to be derived from caring for sick people and then sending them to their homes without food or clothing in their weakened condition," thus the hospital "would be glad to receive more money donations for the work outside the institution." Hall could not "conceive of where a few dollars might be put to better use."[12]

On October 23, Dr. White, city health officer, announced that near-

ly 5,000 Spanish influenza cases had been reported, and at least 400
deaths had resulted from the disease, from the time the epidemic
started in El Paso. There were 229 deaths in the city during the week
ending October 23, an increase of 98 over the previous week. Of the
dead, 144 were Mexican, an increase of 42 over the previous week. An
added explanation of the high death toll among Mexicans was given by
Dr. Tappan. He stated that the "death rate in the Mexican sections that
followed the spread of the influenza epidemic there was due largely to
the fact that there already was an epidemic of whooping cough among
the Mexican children." Tappan commented that "whenever a child
(who is) suffering from that cough is attacked by influenza, the chances
are that the combined attack will prove fatal," and he lamented the
fact that a "good percentage of the deaths on the south side have been
children."[13]

Despite the grim statistics, local interests sometimes objected to the
city's order to close all schools, churches, theatres, and other public
meeting places. However, all requests to reopen them were regretfully
denied. "The epidemic is abating, but has not abated sufficiently to allow reopening," Dr. Tappan declared on October 26. "If we reopened
now," he said, "it would start out again with a whoop." Mayor Davis
agreed, saying: "The health of our people must be given first consideration, and then their financial welfare." But he also said that the "entire
situation should be considered carefully in order that the closing laws
shall not work too great a hardship." However, with 600 deaths so far
in October, the highest fatality rate in the city's history, El Paso's
medical men encouraged "drastic action" to fight the disease. "There is
no use using soft and easy methods at this time if we are going to stamp
out the influenza epidemic," declared city physician White. "We must
get busy and while it may inconvenience us for a while, it will save
lives and much illness in the end." He stated that "it is true the present
orders are working a hardship on certain lines of business here, but the
public health must, and will, be protected." On that note, the board of
health decided that "the lid should be kept tight" regarding the opening
of places in the city. It also ordered "special officers" to help enforce the
rules and regulations for as long as the city remained in "the grip of the
influenza epidemic." They promptly cited several places, including
stores and restaurants, for unnecessary crowding, in spite of the board
of health order that "no stores or public gathering places of any kind,
shall allow more than twenty-five persons other than employees, to
congregate on one floor."[14]

At the same time, in order to help prevent the spread of the disease in houses that already contained flu victims, the Associated Charities increased its "after cure" treatment of patients discharged from Aoy School emergency hospital. The organization's volunteers visited the families of victims in south El Paso, and taught them sanitary and hygienic measures in order to combat a recurrence of the dreaded influenza. Titled "An Ounce of Prevention," a *Times* editorial on October 29, pleaded with the public to abide by the rules and regulations. "There are many people in our community who still need instruction and admonition — in some cases, even severe discipline," and "that is why the rules, rather than relaxed, have been made more rigid."[15]

To make matters worse, the city health inspectors began on October 31 to circulate notices, containing a new military ruling, to "barber shops, soda fountains, soft drink stands, restaurants, fruit and candy stores and the like." It stated that army officers and enlisted men, when given permission to leave Fort Bliss, would be prohibited from patronizing places in El Paso that did not have on display certificates from the board of health stating that "proprietors, employees, and all others who work in the establishment have been examined and found free of communicable diseases." The military had been experiencing a problem with "social diseases" throughout the nation, so at this time it decided to enforce the examination rule in El Paso. Local business and labor interests resented the order, but unless it was followed, local establishments would lose the business of the military.

There were people who considered the military ruling a good idea. A local minister, for example, in a letter to the *Herald*, wrote that "a large number of employees in some of the restaurants have now or have had social diseases in some form." And he declared the following:

> Perhaps I would not be wrong in estimating that seven out of ten have been diseased in that way in the restaurants of which I have knowledge. How do I know that to be true? I have it on the word of the men themselves, cooks, waiters, and others. Most of them are unmarried men and, let me repeat, many of them infected with loathsome diseases. How would you like to have men like that handling meat for you, on a plate, or cutting the bread you eat? Infected persons are also to be found in places other than restaurants. I must heartily endorse, as a result of my own personal knowledge of conditions, the work the authorities are undertaking in regulating health conditions in restaurants, ice cream parlors and other establishments of that nature.[16]

Hundreds of workers volunteered for examinations, but others, especially women, informed the inspectors that they would give up their jobs before submitting to examinations. Mrs. Gertrude Burton, head waitress at the Sheldon Cafe, started a petition drive in protest. Mayor Davis declared that the measure was a "federal government order altogether, deemed necessary for the protection of soldiers." Since it was a military ruling and not a city ordinance, the city could not force anyone to undergo an examination. That would require a city ordinance, and no such ordinance existed. At the same time, Davis noted, the city health department was cooperating by "lending its services" to the military, and therefore those establishments employing workers "not proved free of disease" would be placed "off limits" to servicemen. "The only pressure in the matter," Davis asserted, "would come through the employers who, unless their employees were examined, would lose the trade of the soldiers here." Moreover, added city health officer White, "El Paso has not been imposed upon, for other cities have rigid health examinations for cafes, etc." In fact, he noted that Houston, Dallas, Beaumont, Fort Worth, Galveston, and San Antonio "all have ordinances," and since El Paso did not, it "is necessary for the military to take action."[17]

While the military ruling bemused many El Pasoans, some progress was being made on the flu front. In early November, Dr. White announced that in his opinion the ban could be raised, "as it has been done all over east Texas." The cases "are running low and are not so severe. I feel we can remove the restrictions with safety." Others agreed, and on November 5, during a meeting of Mayor Davis, the city council, and the board of health, a motion was made and passed to lift the health ban on the city and remove the rules and regulations instituted "on account of the prevalence of Spanish influenza." At this time, there were eight cases left in Aoy School emergency hospital, and it no longer functioned in that capacity as soon as those patients were transferred to the county hospital. However, Aoy did reopen as a school for Mexicans, after the building was given a thorough fumigation. Local officials and civic leaders praised the work of the south side institution, and they indicated how its use during the epidemic had illustrated the need for more public health facilities and professionals in El Paso if the city hoped to be adequately prepared to deal with such medical emergencies in the future. For example, Miss A. Louise Dietrich, after thanking the women who helped nurse the sick at the Aoy School emergency hospital during the epidemic, declared that "the work has fully demonstrated to the intelligent public the dire need of a visiting nurses' association, where good nurses may be had for a small sum to care for the sick in their own houses. If such an organization had been in existance here in the past, some of the cases might have been prevented."[18]

On November 6. Dr. White assured the public that the "danger will be passed" by the lifting of the ban on November 9, barring "some unforeseen complication which may arise." Also on November 7, the city council passed a new city ordinance, giving the board of health more power to intervene in case of unforeseen complications. It was considered a farsighted measure that would be good for El Paso. Because of it, noted Mayor Davis, the city should be better prepared to meet deadly epidemics in the future. The new ordinance "empowered the city board of health to adopt any rules and regulations it may deem best to prevent the spread of contagious diseases, and the suppression of same." It required all persons, firms, and corporations to comply with all such orders, and it made all violations punishable by a fine or jail sentence, or both.[19]

El Paso, the "Queen City of the Southwest," reopened on November 9, and the *Times* announced that the "danger for the city as a whole is past and the city will today resume its normal life." It also noted that the board of health urged citizens to continue "individual precautionary measures" in order to prevent a return of the epidemic, along with "the closing of all public entertainments and the prohibition of all public gatherings." The *Herald,* in an editorial entitled "Lifting the Lid," praised the public for its "cheerful cooperation," and stated that because of the measures taken by the city, "thousands of El Paso people owe thanks for their escape from a hard hitting disease and possibly from death." Business and personal privation occurred, noted the paper, but "not once was the fact forgotten that a life means more than money." It also extolled the "devotion" of El Paso's doctors, nurses, and volunteers. Much "unselfish and humanitarian spirit" was exhibited during the crisis.

Also on that day, thousands of people thronged the streets of the business district for the first time in five weeks. With the lifting of the board of health ban on public gatherings, a reporter commented: "The theatres did a rushing business, the stores were kept open until a late hour, and cafes put their jazz bands in operation again." On November 11, El Paso experienced another joyous day. A holiday was declared to celebrate the armistice and the coming of peace in Europe. Over 8,000 people witnessed a "monster parade," and many of them gathered at the El Paso High School stadium and in Pioneer Plaza to hear music and patriotic speeches.[20]

The number of new influenza cases in El Paso suddenly increased following the celebrations, however, health officials did not panic, and by November 18 they observed a gradual decrease. The board of health could not be absolutely sure of the future, but it was believed that the epidemic was definitely on the decline. At that time, the twenty to fifty cases being reported daily were scattered throughout El Paso, and no one section of the city seemed to be suffering more than another. Moreover, on November 24, the quarantine at Fort Bliss was "unconditionally lifted," and hundreds of soldiers who had been confined to the post for eight weeks rushed to El Paso to celebrate. The "Fort Bliss streetcar line was taxed to the limit on incoming trips, especially in the evening," the *Times* observed, as "officers and enlisted men poured into the brightly lighted business district. Shoe shines, shaves and haircuts were obtained on the run, after which many a lad rushed to the home of his·'best girl.'" Taken by surprise, "many a young woman wasn't prepared for the gala event, but nevertheless hasty toilets prepared them for the trip to the movies, dinner at the favorite cafes, or dance parties. Smiling girls and smiling soldiers were numerous."[21]

During the first two weeks of December, daily cases of influenza continued to vary from twenty to forty cases, but from that point on, the number of cases rapidly declined. "The situation here looks mighty good," declared Dr. White on the eve of Christmas, and by the new year the Spanish influenza crisis in El Paso had become history.[22]

In the fall of 1918, the Spanish influenza hit El Paso with devastating force. Although the Texas border community suffered severely, many of its citizens reacted to the crisis in an admirable manner. Individuals and groups in both the public and private sectors worked strenuously to ease the burden brought on by the epidemic. A case in point is the manner in which they joined together to establish the Aoy School emergency hospital to serve the stricken south side of the ciaty. It should also be emphasized that in spite of the dangers, women volunteers — not only in El Paso, but also in the other southwestern cities that suffered from the epidemic — played a major role in combatting the dreaded disease.

❊   ❊   ❊

Chapter III

ALBUQUERQUE

Some Positive Results

% In September 1918, the city of Albuquerque, with a population approaching 15,000, was known as the "metropolis of New Mexico." A regional railroad center located in the rich, irrigated Rio Grande Valley 250 miles north of El Paso, it served a vast area that consisted of farming, ranching, and mining settlements. At that time, Albuquerque was the economic hub of the state, and also the home of the University of New Mexico. In addition, the city had a reputation as a leading health mecca and tourist resort. Promoters referred to it as "Albuquerque, Heart of the Well Country." In September 1918, the newspapers were filled with World War I news, and much of that city's population was engaged in war-related activities. "Pershing Takes 5,000 Prisoners" and "Wilson Urges Support For Fourth Liberty Loan Drive" headlined the local newspapers which also contained occasional reports of the spread of Spanish influenza around the world and the nation. At that time, these latter stories were of lesser interest to Albuquerque citizens.[1]

On October 1, the *Albuquerque Morning Journal* carried a story about the thousands of Spanish influenza cases in Boston, and printed the following instructions on "How to Dodge 'Flu'."

Keep feet and clothing dry.

Avoid crowds.

Protect your nose and mouth in the presence of sneezers.

Gargle your throat three times a day with a mild antiseptic if only salt and water.

Don't neglect a cold.

Keep as much as possible in the sunshine.

Don't get 'scared'.²

On October 5, after eight cases of Spanish influenza, two of them fatal, had been reported to the city physician, the Albuquerque board of health took action. It declared "a state of emergency" in the city, and closed indefinitely all "theatres, churches, schools, both public and private," and prohibited all "public indoor meetings of any kind or character." Local people were urged to take every precaution to prevent the further spread of influenza. They were told to remain as much as possible in their own homes, and to discourage the gathering of people in their houses. They were also told to quickly secure the services of a physician if symptoms of the disease became evident, and to promptly report any death, resulting from the disease, to the city physician.³

On October 7, Dr. E. M. Clayton, city physician, informed the board of health that 75 cases of influenza existed in Albuquerque. Hospitals were filling up with local patients as well as those being sent to Albuquerque from outlying areas. City manager A. R. Hebenstreit issued an order stating that "any person who is ill from any cause" could not enter or leave Albuquerque. At the same time, the University of New Mexico discontinued classes as a health precaution, and Bernalillo county officials followed the lead of Albuquerque officials and announced the closing of all schools and other public meeting places. In the city and county, parents were told to keep children home, and doctors were told to "comply with the ordinance requiring them to acknowledge every case of contagious disease as soon as the diagnosis has been completed." By then, various groups were cancelling conventions scheduled to be held in Albuquerque, and local business and civic leaders wondered what the "health orders" meant for the future of the city. The *Journal*, in an editorial entitled "Don't Let 'Flu' Frighten You To Death," pleaded with them not to panic.⁴

The shortage of nurses was acute. The Red Cross called for volunteers to aid the regular nurses in the hospitals. There was a desperate need for nurses at the University of New Mexico, where the epidemic was severe. On October 13, eight Sisters of Charity, all teachers from the closed St. Vincent's Academy, volunteered to work as nurses at the university. There they looked after the afflicted students, including many "soldier boys" of the Students' Army Training Corps. The Albuquerque *Evening Herald* continued to maintain that there was "no cause for alarm," but by that time there was little doubt that the disease was becoming a serious problem in the city. "The 'FLU' has been the most absorbing topic of interest this week," the *Journal* reported on October 13. Besides "putting a ban on all amusements," (it) has given the teachers and pupils a vacation." And "No one ever before realized what a great part the movies played in the everyday life of Albuquerque." One night during that week, it was reported: "All of the display lights were out and the movies were as dark as a deserted house." One observer said that he "looked for ghosts to appear at any time." Other statements were: "The ghost of fear walked everywhere, causing many a family circle to reunite because of the different members having nothing else to do but stay at home." And: "The Spanish influenza has squelched social activities more effectively than the war and prohibition."[5]

Full page ads began appearing in the newspapers, urging people with influenza symptoms to "Call A Doctor Immediately." "Don't get panicky, but be alert," was the advice of the board of health. On October 17, the board and the city commission, in a joint resolution, banned open-air meetings, and even funeral services were discouraged. The need for strict enforcement of the regulations and for public cooperation was stressed because of the grim statistics. On October 17, George H. Peck, city health officer, reported 394 cases of the disease, with 34 deaths. Those were the "official" statistics. Just two days later the total number of influenza cases reached 489, with 69 deaths.

Meanwhile, the Albuquerque Board of Charities and other benevolent organizations were kept extremely busy during the epidemic. "The work of the Board of Charities has more than doubled," the *Journal* declared. The paper noted that "families which heretofore have not required charitable aid have had their bread winners incapacitated by the disease." Every day "physicians are reporting families which are in dire need of the absolute necessities of life." The Board of Charities received funds from the city government and the Albuquerque Chamber of Commerce, but not enough to meet the demands of the crisis. Organization officials called for more public donations of food, clothing, and money "for the needy who have. been reduced to desperate straits by the influenza." The public response was admirable; not only did people contribute food, clothing, and money, but some of them also volunteered their services to the Board of Charities.[7]

The Spanish influenza epidemic affected the political as well as the social and economic life of Albuquerque. The ban that prohibited indoor and outdoor gatherings was frustrating to politicians, however, for a time it appeared that local political conventions scheduled for late October would indeed be cancelled. One observer suggested that nominations for city and county officers be dispensed with for a year and the present officers be retained. The "ins" found this proposal acceptable, but it was understandably opposed by the "outs." The board of health finally agreed to modify the rules to allow political conventions to meet. The meetings could be held with the understanding that "there be no long speeches, no caucusing, all persons having colds remain at home, and the windows of the convention rooms be left open." The participants complied with these instructions, and the conventions turned out to be short meetings limited to the "bare routine of nominations." The "tamest convention in the history of the Democratic party in Bernalillo County was the one held yesterday at the court house," declared the *Journal* on October 22. The "gathering took on a funeral atmosphere as compared with conventions in the past."[8]

By October 28, a total of 821 cases of Spanish influenza had been reported in Albuquerque. The death count had reached 98, and the board of health once again urged the public to take the "health rules" seriously. It had received complaints from concerned citizens who reported frequent violations of the rules. Particularly upsetting was the "general disposition to ignore influenza quarantine signs entirely, or to regard them lightly." A number of cases were cited "where numbers of families under quarantine have gone about their duties as usual, leaving and entering the house many times a day," or had "torn down signs when they thought the afflicted were cured." The influenza is "worse than Hun bullets," the board declared, and it promised to "get tough" if violations of the rules continued.[9]

The *Journal* pointed out that courageous individuals, such as Sister Alma Louise Vogt of St. Vincent's Academy, had died from influenza while serving as volunteer nurses in Albuquerque, but at the same time other individuals were breaking the "health rules." It was difficult, however, to persuade the entire population to follow instructions. For example, religious groups flooded city officials with requests to resume church services, but the officials remained adamant in their stand that "the lid be kept on for the present." As they viewed it, the influenza epidemic had "not improved to the extent that it would be wise to relax the health rules in the least." They stated that other cities had "raised the lid" only to be compelled to replace it in a few days. "It is the firm intention of city authorities to keep the epidemic under control," the *Herald* declared, "and they should be commended for their action." Yet it was difficult to enforce the rules all of the time. On holidays, for example, the temptation to celebrate was difficult to resist. On November

3, a *Journal* editor wrote that "Albuquerque society is as dead — almost — as the proverbial 'door nail.' Of course the lid was tilted slightly on Halloween and a few parties were attended by the younger set, despite the rulings of the board of health."[10]

By November 6, five weeks after the epidemic had begun in Albuquerque, the "official" number of influenza cases reported in the city reached 923; of which a total of 167 had died. The hospitals were still crowded, and the resources of the charitable organizations were increasingly strained. Local residents continued to volunteer their services to care for those who needed help. The Albuquerque Board of Charities operated an emergency hospital for the destitute at their "colony" located at Third Street and Mountain Road. The "best care possible was administered to patients who had no place to turn for assistance when stricken with the disease, as all hospitals in the city were filled to capacity," noted the *Herald*. The Board of Charities also sent its representatives into the homes of the sick. In one instance, reported the paper, "a widow woman with five children died after an attack of Spanish influenza. Several of the children are sick. There are four girls, aged 2, 6, 10, and 14, and a boy of 8 years. They had little food or clothing. They are being looked after by the board and homes will be found for them."[11]

While expressions of appreciation for the endeavors of physicians, nurses, and welfare workers were frequently heard, others also made sacrifices. As in other cities, essential services suffered in Albuquerque. Fire and police departments lost members, while streetcar and telephone companies lost operators. For example, the *Journal* mentioned the local telephone operators who played an important role in the relief work for Spanish influenza victims. "Patient, tired little girls, for such they really were in many cases, crowded into service before their full term of instruction was completed," the newspaper stated, "willingly working overtime to relieve a sister worker who had the flu, struggling with excited patrons who spoke English imperfectly or called wrong numbers, doing double the work by day and night that would have been required of them in normal times. Surely a vote of thanks is due these 'soldiers of the switchboard.'"

Despite the health rules, Albuquerque joined the region and the nation in celebrating the end of World War I. Practically the whole city turned out to "make merry," noted the *Journal*. It observed that Albuquerqueans, "regardless of age, nationality, or sex, joined almost as a unit in giving vent to their feelings of joy over the signing of the armistice by the Germans." A huge parade started at Central Avenue and Second Street and moved west on Central to Robinson Park, and to the *Journal*, it "seemed to be an endless chain of cheering, howling humanity." According to the *Herald*, "the twenty odd thousand residents of this town who were able to get out of bed or leave the baby or their job mingled together on the downtown streets in greater numbers and closer contact than for many years." The people "raised great clouds of dust and joyously and fearlessly breathed it in. They didn't think of dust, or of the germs it might contain." During the celebration, "they didn't think of Spanish influenza or any other variety of bugs." Here then, the paper declared, "is a fair test of the contagious character of this new-fangled kind of grippe. If, within the next forty-eight hours there should be a large increase in the number of cases of 'flu' in Albuquerque we will know that quarantine and the orders against ordinary activities and assemblages is right." On the other hand, "if we emerge from our splendid orgy of Thanksgiving without any such serious consequence, we will know that we have been suffering to some extent from fright during the past several weeks — and that it's time to lift the quarantine and get back to normal."[12]

Since the influenza crisis had not intensified by November 15, on that date the city commission and the board of health agreed to lift the quarantine and other restrictions if the epidemic did not worsen. "It was deemed advisable to allay the fears of the people along this line as much as possible," the *Journal* asserted, for "the idea of those in authority all along has been to restore normal conditions just as soon as possible." The paper emphasized that at no time had there been a disposition on the part of the members of the city commission or the board of health "to keep schools, churches, lodges, movie shows and other places of assembly closed any longer than was thought necessary."[13]

At the same time, according to Rabbi Moise Bergman, secretary of the Albuquerque Board of Charities, the number of influenza cases was on the increase "among the poor in the city," and the demands being made upon his organization were more intense than at any other time during the epidemic. Bergman knew what he was talking about. A *Journal* reporter accompanied him on his rounds on November 20, and declared that "unless you had seen it you could scarcely believe that within the borders of Albuquerque there existed such absolute squalor." They "visited a back room of an old adobe house on Tijeras Avenue, and beheld there an ancient iron bed, whose broken and sagging springs allowed the thin and dirty mattress to touch the floor under the weight of a human shape which lay upon it, covered partly by a poor torn piece of what was once a comforter." The "form under the torn quilt proved to be that of an old colored man, a paralytic, who for months had been occupying this same bed and has been depending upon the generosity of whoever came along that he could ask for a drink of water or a bite of food." Rabbi Bergman told the reporter that he could show him "several others, most of them white, who are in practically as destitute a condition." Bergman also informed the *Journal* representative that "we are doing the best we can, as fast as these cases come to our notice, to either move them out of their squalid surroundings or to improve them, but the city hospital is overcrowded with indigent flu cases and our finances are not unlimited."

Rabbi Bergman led the drive to raise $10,000 for the poor in Albuquerque. He noted that the "demands for funds is more urgent than ever this year due to the fact that the epidemic of influenza through which Albuquerque has passed during the last two months has produced conditions with which those in charge of the city's charities have never had to contend in the past." He pointed out that "many children have been left orphans." In many cases, "husbands and fathers have been taken away, leaving little hungry mouths to feed and frail bodies to clothe." In other cases, "mothers have entered upon 'the sleep that knows no waking,' leaving fathers, who in many cases have had Spanish influenza and were kept away from their work for weeks, to care for small children." In fact, Bergman concluded, "the exigencies of the situation call for greater liberality than ever before on the part of those who can afford to give." Bergman also supported the city commission and the board of health in opposing the requests of critics to open up Albuquerque before December 1. As he put it, city officials "have been level-headed and I admire their stand. I also think that the quarantine should by all means be made more stringent until the disease is entirely wiped out." He admitted that "it is hard to answer the man who says his business has been hurt by the restrictions, but it will be impossible to answer the one who says 'my child has died because of the neglect of the city.'"[14]

City fathers insisted on keeping the lid on in Albuquerque; they did not want to make the mistake of officials in Denver and other cities. "Some people in Albuquerque advocate the premature lifting of the ban in this city," the *Journal* declared, but "do they want Albuquerque to experience Denver's serious situation?" A long article followed describing how "premature" action in opening up Denver had resulted in a renewal of the Spanish influenza epidemic in that city. The *Herald* also noted the unfortunate Denver experience, and commended local authorities for learning from it. It reported that "the board of health and the city commission have turned a deaf ear to the requests of a number of people that the Spanish flu ban be lifted before December 1." The requests "come mainly from those who are speaking from a financial standpoint." City officials pointed out that it remained their "highly important duty to stand guard to protect the interests of the people at large and not to permit anything to be done, that in the opinion of the best informed medical men in the country, will jeopardize the life and health of the community."

City officials in Albuquerque realized that many people were suffering a severe financial loss during the ban period. Against this loss, they cited the fact that since the onset of the epidemic in that city, hundreds of Spanish influenza cases, many of them fatal, had been reported. They noted "the widows and orphans, and broken hearts; people of all ages and classes left in destitute circumstances, in many instances, because of the unforeseen taking away of some member of a family." "We dislike very much to continue the ban," stated a member of the board of health, but "the complaints that we hear in regard to the ban are mainly from people whose pocketbooks have been hit." "We do not desire any person to lose money," he remarked, "but in this situation we must consider the community as an entirety and do what we believe to be best for the good of everybody concerned."[15]

After interviewing a number of Albuquerqueans, a *Journal* reporter observed that views of the subject ran the gamut. Some believed the restrictions to be "entirely useless," while others called for "more stringent" restrictions, including the wearing of masks. Most of those interviewed agreed with city officials. Indeed, when comments began to increase, concerning an election to recall city commissioners if they did not lift the ban, the local press discouraged it. "They have done nothing to merit recall," the *Journal* declared, and it concluded that, as a result of the restrictions, Albuquerque had suffered less than many cities of comparable size.[16]

The restrictions were continued until the city commissioners considered it safe enough to lift the ban and finally, on November 28, 1918, the *Herald* announced that the "Spanish influenza has spent its force on Albuquerque," and that the city could resume normal activities on December 1. New public health provisions, such as "trained nurses" in the schools and "regular inspections" of public places, would be observed, and a return to normal was expected. On that date, a Sunday, Albuquerqueans crowded into the churches and theatres. As the *Journal* put it, "people were as frisky as a flock of colts just turned out to pasture in the early spring after being held in restraint during the winter months." M. P. Williamson, owner of the Ideal Theatre, spoke for many local commercial interests when he stated that his place had the "biggest business day in its history," and he noted that he "had never seen more appreciative audiences."[17]

In the week following the lifting of the ban, an increase in the number of Spanish influenza cases occurred, but local officials did not take any new action. They continued to urge individuals to take vaccine and other precautionary measures, but the *Journal* announced that "wild rumors about restoring the influenza ban are without foundation." Indeed, on December 6, the *Herald* declared that "Albuquerque society is frolicking once more." On December 16, the board of health stated that the influenza epidemic was no worse than it had been under the ban. It also noted that the "cases reported now are not as serious as they were at first."[18]

At the same time, the board of health supported the establishment of a state department of health in New Mexico " to afford the protection, which has hitherto been accorded animals, plant life, and other property, but has been denied human beings." Of all the southwestern states, New Mexico was the only one without a state department of health, and this fact became a source of embarrassment to enlightened Albuerqueans during the Spanish influenza epidemic. The need for such an agency aroused a great deal of interest in the "metropolis of New Mexico." For example, at a meeting sponsored by the Albuquerque Chamber of Commerce on December 18, city officials from throughout the state formed the New Mexico League of Cities. The urban leaders discussed various problems facing New Mexico's cities, and they all agreed that a definite need existed, especially after hearing a speech by John Tombs, secretary of the New Mexico Public Health Association. Tombs disclosed that in 1916 the president of the American Public Health Association had investigated public health conditions in the Southwest, and concluded that "New Mexico sells health but does not know whether she herself is healthy or not." Tombs also cited a report compiled by a national commission in which a prominent physician made the following observation regarding New Mexico: "It is unfortunate that a state with a population that numbers nearly half a million should do so little for public health." After listening to Tombs, the League of Cities issued a statement proclaiming it "a pleasure to endorse a state department of health in New Mexico."[19]

The New Mexico Public Health Association met often in Albuquerque during the winter and spring months of 1918-1919, and it always urged the creation of an effective and properly financed state department of health by the New Mexico legislature. On January 8, 1919 the *Herald* declared Albuquerque to be in "total sympathy with the drive to secure New Mexico from the menace of health ignorance." A week later O. A. Larrazolo, governor of New Mexico, pleaded with the incoming state legislature to create a state department of health with broad powers and asked for an ample amount of money in order to carry out its duties. As he put it, "it is needless for me to point out to you the crying demand and undeniable necessity for the creation and maintenance of such a department." The "terrible ravages made among our people, and throughout the nation at large, by reason of the epidemic of influenza, made us all open our eyes to the great mistake that we have made in not making proper provision for the meeting of such destructive visitations." In turn, on March 14, the New Mexico legislature officially established a state department of health. It was created to serve as "the superior health authority of the state" and it was given "the power to investigate, control and abate the causes of disease, especially epidemics." Reformers throughout the state and the nation considered the birth of the new agency a "progressive step in the right direction."[20]

Meanwhile, Albuquerque had returned to normal. Although no substantial increase in the number of Spanish influenza cases occurred during the holiday season, the city did experience a "flare-up" that exceeded 100 cases during a four day period in late January, 1919. However, by February 10 the *Herald*, noting that not a single new case of the disease had been reported within 72 hours, was pleased to announce that in Albuquerque "the flu has flew."[21]

As was the case in El Paso, the Spanish influenza epidemic brought untold suffering to Albuquerque in the fall of 1918, and the crisis produced a broad-based community response to combat the disease. The Albuquerque experience also illustrated the crucial role of volunteers in dealing with the problem. Courageous individuals like Sister Alma Louise Vogt and Rabbi Moise Bergman served as outstanding examples of personal involvement and community leadership. Furthermore, the people of Albuquerque, individually and collectively, while responding to the needs created by the epidemic, played an influential role in promoting new local and state health regulations designed to serve as future preventative measures. In neighboring Arizona, community response to the "flu invasion" was equally evident, but the nature of the effort was different.

※   ※   ※

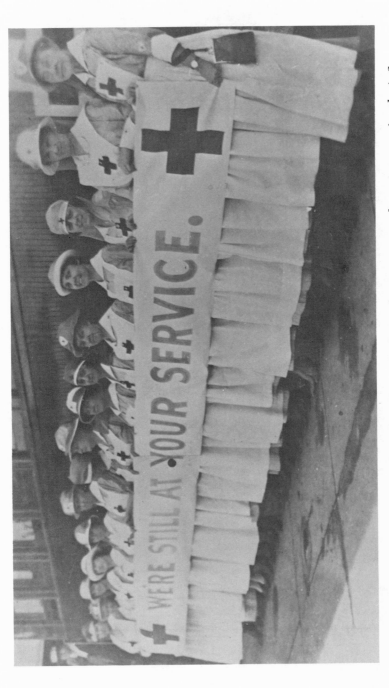

In El Paso, the Red Cross contributed medicines, beds for the patients, and nursing care for the influenza victims. Shown above are some of the Red Cross workers.

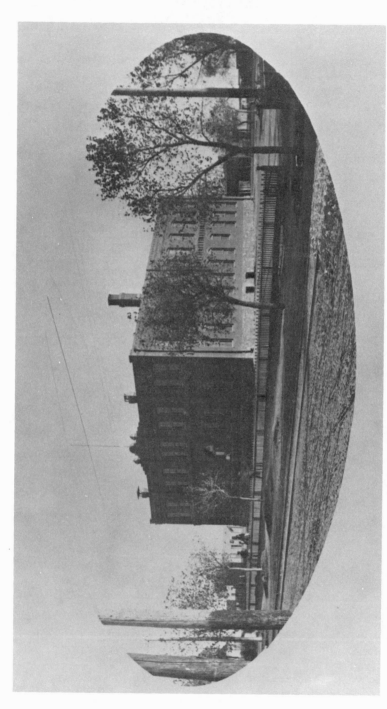

Aoy School in South El Paso was converted into an emergency hospital during the epidemic, where care was pro-vided for influenza patients, particularly those from that area of the city.

COURTESY EL PASO PUBLIC LIBRARY

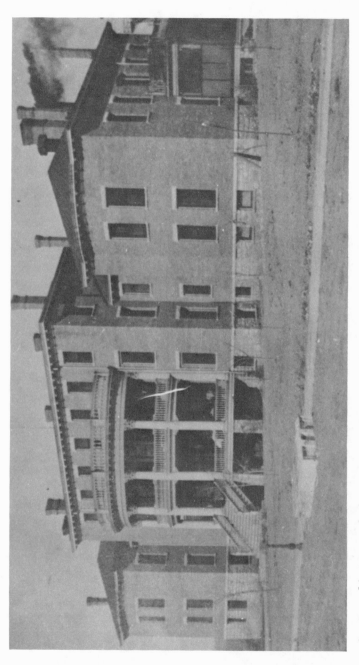

St. Joseph's Hospital, as it was in 1918. Like the other hospitals in Albuquerque during the influenza epidemic, it was filled to capacity with flu victims. COURTESY ALBUQUERQUE MUSEUM PHOTOARCHIVES

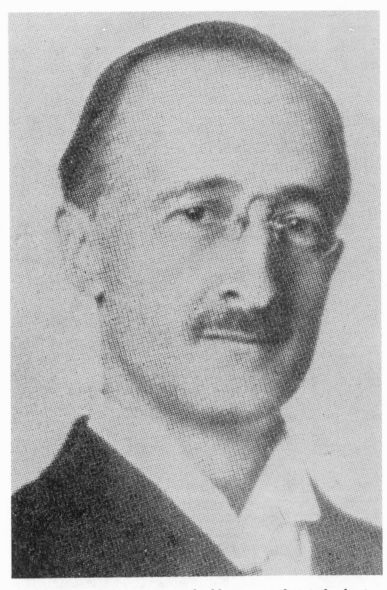

Rabbi Moise Bergman was a highly respected civic leader in the community of Albuquerque and one of the leaders in the effort to provide aid and comfort to the many influenza victims during the 1918 epidemic. Courtesy Albuquerque Elks Club

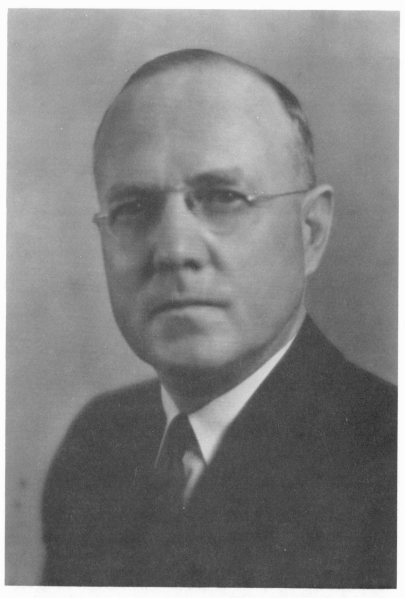

Dr. Meade Clyne was one of the Tucson City Health Officers who contributed much time and effort in attempting to contain the influenza epidemic in the community.

COURTESY ARIZONA HISTORICAL SOCIETY

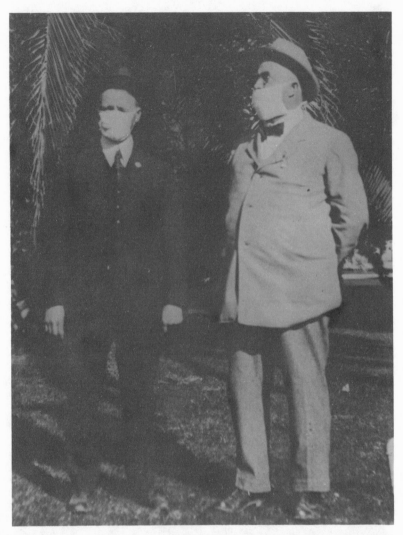

In 1918 during the influenza epidemic, Arizona Governor W.P. Hunt (right) and C.M. Zander, chairman of the Arizona State Tax Commission, were photographed wearing their "flu" masks, in accordance with the regulations at that time. The above photo appeared in the December 8, 1918 issue of the Arizona Republican. *The number of sharp-eyed readers who noticed that the Governor was not wearing his mask correctly is not known.*

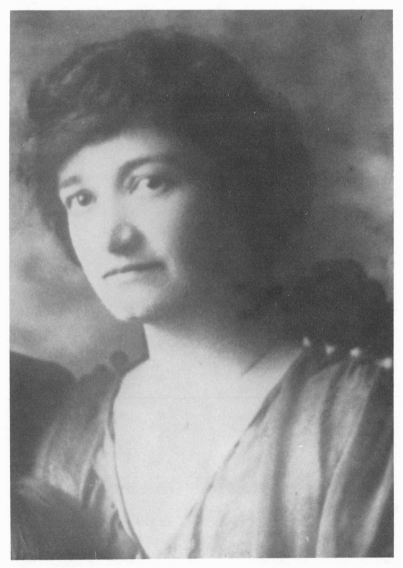

During the 1918 flu epidemic, Mrs. Baron Goldwater (mother of Barry Goldwater) was supervisor of the Red Cross women of Phoenix who provided the Women's Club emergency hospital with a variety of goods, including clothing and bedding.

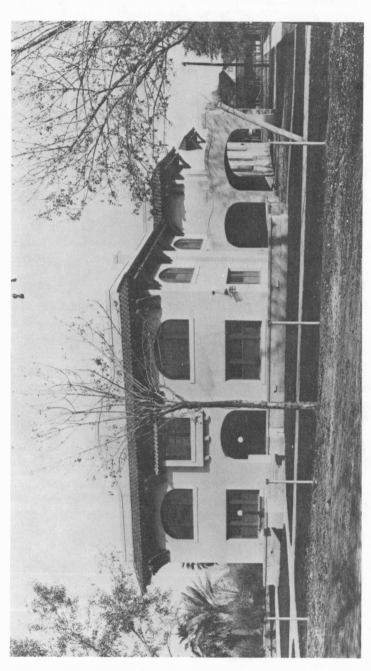

The Phoenix Women's Club was temporarily converted into an emergency hospital during the 1918 flu epidemic, in order to provide care and treatment for those stricken by the disease.

Chapter IV

TUCSON

To Mask Or Not To Mask

꙾꙾ Tucson, advertised as a city "where winter never comes" by the
꙾꙾ Southern Pacific Railroad and other promoters, had a population of some 18,000 people in 1918. It enjoyed a national reputation as
a health haven and tourist attraction. It also served as a leading trade
and distribution center in the region. The University of Arizona,
located in the city, was recognized as the cultural hub of the state. In
September 1918, the newspapers of Tucson, as in other cities, were full
of war stories, with only occasional items about the spread of Spanish
influenza around the country.[1]

By early October, no cases of Spanish influenza had been reported in
Tucson, but detailed items regarding the effects of the epidemic
elsewhere were appearing in the local press on a regular basis. Some
Tucson residents expressed fear, and the *Arizona Daily Star* warned
them not to catch "Spanish hysteria." As Dr. Meade Clyne, city health
officer, declared on October 5, "Tucson so far has been passed up by
the influenza germs and there is no cause for alarm." At the same time.
R. B. Von Kleinsmed, president of the University of Arizona, placed
the school under quarantine as a preventative measure. The War
Department, concerned about the health of members of the Students'
Army Training Corps at the University, had issued orders to the school
to take every precaution. Von Kleinsmed told the *Tucson Citizen* that
"no cases of Spanish influenza have developed on campus and none in
the city so far as known, but that University authorities desire to see if
the campus cannot be kept free from the epidemic."[2]

Within the next several days, Spanish influenza hit Arizona hard. On
October 10, two dozen cases were reported in Tucson, and Dr. Clyne
received a telegram from Dr. Orville Harry Brown, state superintend-

[29]

ent of public health, instructing him on how to handle the situation. Brown, acting on the advice of Surgeon General Rupert Blue of the United State Public Health Service, advised Clyne that "all places of public gatherings" should be closed. Brown also urged Clyne to ask all physicians in the Tucson area to report influenza cases immediately, and to see that strict quarantine measures be carried out with those infected. Local newspapers were requested to publish tips on "How To Guard Against The Spanish Influenza" such as the following:

Avoid contact with other people as far as possible.

Avoid persons suffering with colds, sore throats, and coughs.

Avoid chilling the body or getting overheated.

Sleep and work in clean, fresh air.

Keep hands clean and keep them out of the mouth.

Avoid spitting in public places.

Eat plain, nourishing food.

Cover the nose with handkerchief when you sneeze, the mouth when
   you cough. Change handkerchiefs frequently.

If you get a cold, go to bed in a well-ventilated room.

Avoid kissing.

If you get the influenza, go to bed and call the best physician you can afford.

Don't worry.[3]

The first cases of Spanish influenza to develop in Tucson were found chiefly among the railroad men who worked on the trains in and around the Southern Pacific facilities. The disease soon moved out into the general population, affecting in particular the Mexican section "south of the tracks." As the number of cases increased in the city, the medical men, led by Dr. Clyne, met to consider the advice of Drs. Blue and Brown. After pooling their observations, they recommended that a strict quarantine be established. On October 10, Mayor O. C. Parker issued an order closing the schools, churches, theatres, and all "other places where people congregate." The police were instructed to prevent crowds from gathering in the city streets. The mission San Xavier del Bac was closed to tourists, the Carnegie Library shut its doors, and classes at the University of Arizona were suspended.[4]

By October 17, there were 120 cases of Spanish influenza in the city and another 100 cases at the University of Arizona. City hospitals were filled with patients and an emergency hospital had been improvised in the University gymnasium to care for afflicted students. Some institutions were especially hard hit. For example, the Tucson Indian Training School, four miles south of the city, reported 130 cases of the disease on October 24. Only ten students at the school did not have the disease. The "Mexican quarter of the city, where houses are poorly ventilated," continued to have more than its share of cases. The *Star* felt that the conditions and the number of victims in the Mexican barrios emphasized the importance of good sanitation and ventilation as preventative measures.[5]

While local editorial writers were advising the public to "keep cool," and follow the rules and regulations, they also called for more volunteer doctors and nurses to meet the crisis. At the same time, news of World War I dominated the papers. Headlines announcing the decisive role being played by Americans in the conflict appeared daily, and Tucson was ready to celebrate when news of the armistice reached the city. A holiday atmosphere prevailed on November 11, while the "greatest celebration in the history of Tucson" took place. Despite the rules and regulations, flag-waving crowds paraded the streets and sidewalks of the city. The police kept busy trying to keep order. People danced around bonfires that blazed in the central part of town. At times "the celebration on Congress Street approached a riot," declared the *Star*, "owing to the use of tin cans and fire crackers."[6]

Complaints could be heard in towns and cities throughout the state from individuals and groups that were adversely affected by the official efforts to curb the epidemic. Especially vocal were the owners of business establishments whose profits depended on customers in their stores. However, those connected to religious and educational institutions also expressed criticism. On November 14, the state board of health outlined seven points as preliminary requisites to the reopening of public places in a community. The board noted that it would give permission to local health officials to lift bans once the points were met, providing the epidemic was on the decrease in the area. The seven points made a formidable list:

1. There must be a universal, thorough cleaning of streets, alleys, yards and other places needing same.
2. A thorough scrubbing with hot water and soap, or other approved method of cleaning, of all buildings, schools, churches, theatres, and other places where public meetings are held.
3. Placards for display must be printed and distributed to houses where influenza patients are located.

4. Conspicuous posters must be put prominently in all public places, calling attention to the dangers of coughing, sneezing, spitting, hand-shaking, and kissing, the use of dishes, glasses, and other tableware which have not been thoroughly washed in hot water since their previous use.

5. Inspection must be made by competent persons appointed by local health officers to ascertain if the food and drinking places are giving proper attention to the washing of their dishes and glasses, and other utensils used in the preparation and serving of food and drink.

6. Receptacles must be placed upon the streets at such places and in such numbers as may be necessary to serve as sputum basins. A prominent sign should be placed over each receptacle, calling attention to the necessity of spitting in the receptacle and not upon the sidewalk or street or other inappropriate place.

7. An effort must be made to induce everybody to take the influenza vaccine. This effort must be honest, serious and systematic.

The seven points were printed in the *Star* and the *Citizen* in Tucson, and soon progress in meeting the points was evident, "so far as practicable." Local health officials, including Dr. Clyne, asserted that "the general sanitation of the city" was good, but they also declared that "since the further condition imposed by the state board, that the epidemic must be on the decrease, is not true at Tucson, action is automatically deferred." Dr. Brown, on behalf of the state board of health, agreed with the decision of the Tucson medical men, and in a telegram to Dr. Clyne advised him and his colleagues not to reopen the city.[7]

On November 16, the number of cases reported in Tucson rose to 18, up from 10 the previous day. Some observers believed that the crowds that participated in the armistice celebration had stimulated the spread of the disease. The *Star* urged the public to abide by the rules and regulations. It also suggested a mask order might be the answer. At certain points on the Pacific coast the "use of the gauze mask has come much into favor." In San Francisco its "use was enforced and as a result the city was opened." Many believed that the citizens of Tucson should follow the example of the California city. The use of the mask "can do no harm," it was said, and "it may do a great deal of good." It was urged that the city health officer issue an order "to the effect that every man, woman and child in Tucson wear a mask."[8]

On November 17, Dr. Clyne called together the city board of health to consider the Spanish influenza situation, and it was decided that not enough progress was being made in combating the disease. It was also decided that "masks should be worn in any place where people meet for the transaction of necessary business." In addition, the order stated that owners of business establishments "shall not, at any time, permit more than one customer to every 500 square feet of floor space," and it prohibited loitering in the stores or streets. To encourage participation, the order stated that violators of the new rules and regulations would be punished by a fine of not less than ten dollars, or by imprisonment for a term not exceeding thirty days, or by both fine and imprisonment.[9]

Following the issuance of the order, the local Red Cross sent out a call for workers to report to its headquarters and prepare a large supply of masks, for use by the general public. Although the volunteer workers made 2300 masks in twenty-four hours, more were needed. The Red Cross found that the demand for the masks far exceeded the supply. More women volunteered and more masks were made. The "biggest crowd in the city was before the Red Cross shop waiting to buy masks," declared the *Citizen*. They were "snatched up as quickly as manufactured by the women inside." Of course the crowd rule was being violated, but "the doors were locked to keep out the public." And so it went. The "official" flu mask "covered the nose and mouth and consisted of at least four thicknesses of butter cloth or at least seven thicknesses or ordinary gauze." The Red Cross also emphasized that the masks proved "worse than useless" if they were not frequently sterilized.

New styles in anti-germ masks appeared almost simultaneously with the issuance of the order. The *Star* noted that "the public will be offered, no doubt, positively the latest thing in masks." The *Citizen* described "a nifty California mask" which conformed to the shape of the nose. It "is made by taking a square of cloth, folded as many thicknesses as desired, 11 by 13 inches, nicking two of the corners and sewing up the slits so as to make a shallow bag. Strings or ear loops are sewed off the other corners. The strings may be tied over the top of the head." For the most part, declared the paper, the "inconvenience of the mask was taken good-naturedly, and there was even much hilarity over the large numbers of 'highwaymen' in the city."[10]

But was it working? By November 20, twenty cases of influenza a day were being reported in Tucson. On that date, police began to make arrests, if necessary, in efforts to enforce the masking order. As chief of police Frank Bailey put it: "All persons seen entering places of business without masks adjusted over nose and mouth will be taken into custody, in compliance with the order which has the effect of law

within the city limits." Bailey also stated that the "lack of a requirement that masks be worn on the street makes enforcement of the order
difficult for the police, but they will do the best they can."

Enforcement of the rules and regulations was a problem, and it
bothered a number of individuals and groups. "Generally, people are
observing the masking order," Dr. Clyne asserted on November 21, but
"enforcement continues to be by propaganda instead of by penalty of
the law." Therefore the public "does not fear arrest." He reiterated his
faith in the mask as a method of combating Spanish influenza, and he
called upon the public to support the board of health in its effort to do
something effective towards controlling the disease. As for the enforcement of the masking order, he declared that "he could not see to it
because that duty devolved upon the police and the chief of police was
derelict in his duty in this respect." Groups of merchants complained
that unmasked persons entered stores "at every minute of the day."
They stated that if masking could stamp out the epidemic quickly then
it should be "carried to the limit." They also took the position that they
could not be expected to police their stores against unmasked persons.
That should be the duty of the police, but "the chief has indicated by
his failure to enforce the penalty for the violation of the masking order
that he prefers to use the method of solicitation." The merchants believed that if the mask order were rigidly enforced, an early lifting of
the ban might be expected. Time and again, they used the San Francisco experience to make their point.[11]

To meet the criticism and to encourage the enforcement of the masking order, the board of health on November 22 issued an amendment to
the original order stating that "no person shall appear in any street,
park, place where any business is transacted, or in any other public
place within the city of Tucson, without wearing a mask consisting of
at least four thicknesses of butter cloth or at least seven thicknesses of
ordinary gauze, covering both the nose and the mouth." The order
affected children as well as adults, and parents were held responsible
for their children. The amendment, declared the *Star*, "requires
universal, unconditional wearing of masks in Tucson." The "only exception is the privacy of one's own home." To help enforce the amendment, Mayor Parker appointed twenty-five "special non-uniformed
policemen" to assist in the proper enforcement of the order.[12] (The purpose of using non-uniformed police was so they could easily spot those
who were not conforming to the mask-wearing amendment, before

those non-conformists spotted them and then had time to quickly and only temporarily don the masks).

By Thanksgiving Day, an unmasked face was a rare sight in Tucson. On that day, however, the spiritual hardship caused by the denial of religious services was evident. Dr. J. B. Brown of the Christian Church had asked Dr. Clyne if the churches could open if the congregation were masked, but the city health officer replied that they could not, nor could he say when they would be allowed to open the places of worship. Clergymen were disappointed in not being able to meet with their congregations, but the *Citizen* offered to make itself "the medium of messages from pastors to their flocks, thus supplying in a measure the loss of the service of the day." The sermons subsequently printed in the paper were much appreciated.

By this time, the number of influenza cases in Tucson had declined. Observers noted a significant improvement since the increase of the disease resulting from the victory celebration, and they wondered if the time had arrived to open up the city. The *Citizen* stated: "With the announcement that for some time there have been only six new cases of influenza in Tucson daily, it would seem that there is no good reason for keeping the city closed up tight, particularly in view of the fact that the masking order is being universally enforced. It would be interesting to know whether, with six new cases a day, the authorities will tie Tucson up all winter." Thinking of the effect of the disease on the economy, the paper asked "what is to be the limit. Must the city be entirely free from the influenza or any old cold that can be construed as such before the ban is lifted?" If Tucson business interests "could know when the quarantine now being enforced will end, they could better weather the storm." The *Citizen* declared: "The only thing that is holding back the big expansion in business expected at the close of the war here in southern Arizona is the quarantine." On Saturday, November 30, it suggested that the health authorities do the "sensible thing and open up Tucson early next week.[13]

Others agreed with the editors of the *Citizen*, and the pressure was on. Dr. Clyne, after a telephone conversation with Dr. Brown, the state health officer, called the local board of health together on December 1 to discuss the situation, and it agreed to lift the influenza quarantine, but retain the masking order. This meant that the theatres could reopen, but only those wearing masks would be admitted. Churches could resume services, but members of the congregation had to wear masks. In business establishments, proprietors, clerks, and customers were still required to be masked. Persons in any place where people congregated were also required to wear them. In short, the new order did not "discard" masks, and "careful citizens" were urged to keep carrying them. Schools, however, were exempt from the modified order. Dr. Clyne explained it was because of the new seating arrangement in the schools, whereby three feet of space was kept between pupils at all times. They occupied every other desk in the rooms and were required to keep their distance from each other at all times during school hours. This was made possible by splitting the student population into morning and afternoon sessions to limit crowded conditions. Another reason for exempting school children from wearing the masks, Clyne said, was that "they appear not to be very susceptible to the disease."[14]

The quarantine had been in effect since October 10, and for fifty-one days local businesses had been hit hard. With some of the restrictions lifted, it was time to celebrate. The "lid is off" declared the *Citizen*. Merchants held big sales, and the stores were crowded. Clerks had a difficult time waiting on all the customers. Automobiles lined the curbs of the business district, and pedestrians filled the streets and sidewalks. Crowds of "starved movie fans came down on the theatres with one grand rush." Early Christmas buyers came out in force, and the Tucson newspaper, the *Star*, reported that the "holiday business promises to be unprecedented." With the lifting of the ban, local leaders expected "a big influx of winter visitors." Altogether, the *Citizen* asserted, "Tucson is expected to put on the busiest appearance in its history and to enter upon a long season of prosperity held back at the coming of the armistice by the quarantine."

Although the "lifting of the lid" did not mean the lifting of the masks, a disappointed Dr. Clyne stated that the masking order was being "utterly ignored." He urged enforcement of the "modified order" to prevent a "second visitation of the influenza epidemic upon the city." He reminded the public that since the first epidemic visited Tucson, the city had experienced 650 cases of Spanish influenza, resulting in 70 deaths. Clyne mentioned a recent American Medical Association report which emphasized that organization's belief in "the efficacy of the mask." He pointed out that when the masks came off too soon in a number of other cities, including San Francisco, a second epidemic had occurred. Chief Bailey admitted that enforcement was difficult, if not lax, however he warned that "if the modified order is abused and the epidemic breaks out again, the original closing order, possibly with radical amendments, will be invoked again." He believed the public wanted to avoid that experience, and he said: "It is certainly in the interests of those businessmen and others affected by the closing order to cooperate with us in the enforcement of the mask order."

On December 13, the Tucson city council passed a new ordinance that required masks to be worn. The mask ordinance simply required what the existing board of health masking order required, but it gave more force to the edict. Dr. Clyne expressed his satisfaction, and Chief Bailey pledged to enforce the new ordinance; indeed, he reminded city council members that it would be well for them to "provide themselves with masks." Mayor Parker also promised to cooperate. He even suggested that Chief Bailey send a policeman into each of the city churches on Sunday to see that the ordinance was being obeyed. "It won't hurt a policeman to go into church once," he observed. The press supported the measure to a degree. The *Star* urged compliance with the mask ordinance in order to prevent another epidemic. The *Citizen* was hesitant, but willing to go along. "We never thought much of the masking business," it said, but since the people "have delegated to certain authorities the power to make regulations on these matters and if they order us to mask, the only thing to do is submit gracefully whether or not we have any confidence in the little rag which they ask us to wear over our noses." The "fellow who does not believe in the mask should be willing to wear it for the peace of mind of the fellow who does."[15]

Scores of arrests followed the issuance of the mask ordinance. "We are going to enforce this ordinance or close up the town entirely," declared Chief Bailey. On December 18, forty-six persons were cited by the police for failure to wear masks and were ordered to report to hearings before Judge L. O. Cowan in the city court. The *Citizen*, suggesting "The Law of Masking" needed more precise definition, noted that "an entirely new jurisprudence is being built up and lawyers who do not familiarize themselves with it will be behind the times." It would be in order for Judge L. O. Cowan of Tucson, "who is deciding the important questions arising in these cases to give us a work on the subject so that the coming generation of lawyers may use it as a textbook for the law of masking." In the future, an attorney's education would be incomplete without knowledge of this subject, the *Citizen* predicted, for "how is one to know what constitutes a violation unless he is familiar with the many rulings on the subject."

On the day before the *Citizen* editorial appeared, Judge Cowan had found eight persons guilty of violations of the masking ordinance, and they had eight different excuses. "If the experience of the eight persons serves as an example of what to expect," the *Citizen* wrote, then "the authority who compiles a summary of the decisions will be performing a public service." In short, "there must be some definition of the term 'masked' worked out so that all may know what constitutes a proper adjustment of the little rag."

Judge Cowan, in finding the eight persons guilty of failing to wear anti-germ masks, had made a start in interpreting the city ordinance, but his decisions left the *Citizen* puzzled. The decisions in the cases, as they appeared in the paper, follow:

City of Tucson vs. S. Kogas —
The defendant in this case is the proprietor of a fruit stand open at the front. He wore his mask over his mouth, but not over his nose. Held by Judge Cowan that a recent operation on the nose which makes it difficult to breathe through a mask is no defense. Also that the fact a Greek is 12,000 miles from home, has lived in California eight years, has never before been jerked up before a court, tries to pay his debts and his rent, and is otherwise of good moral character, does not entitle defendant to remission of fine.

City of Tucson vs. Antonio Gutierrez —
The defendant in this case is delivery man for the S. P. Grocery. Claimed that he was busy loading groceries in box and did not hear policeman tell him to put mask on. Held by Judge Cowan that defendant was not entitled to a second warning before arrest.

City of Tucson vs. Louis P. Cota —
Defendant in this case is a window washer employed at the White House Cafe. Wore mask over chin. Held by Judge Cowan that window washer may not remove mask from mouth for purpose of blowing on window panes in order to dry them.

City of Tucson vs. J. Simon —
Defendant is employee of pool room. Held by Judge Cowan that person engaged in racking the balls may not remove mask while so engaged. Defendant entered exceptions after being fined on ground under 16 years of age, and fine remitted. Case transferred to juvenile court.

City of Tucson vs. Pierre I. Rally —
Defendant in this case lives in rear of store and was engaged in cleaning showcase. Held by Judge Cowan that front part of store was a place of business, rear was residence, and that defendant must wear mask while engaged in cleaning out showcase, even when alone in store.

City of Tucson vs. J. Calisher —
Defendant claimed he had been out of town and didn't know that mask
order was being enforced again. Hates to pay out week's wages for
brief privilege of fresh air. Held by Judge Cowan that ignorance of the
law is no excuse, after a person has been warned by a policeman.
City of Tucson vs. S. Simon —
Defendant had just thrown cigar away and was about to replace mask.
Does not think it necessary to wear one when few customers are
around. Held by Judge Cowan that inconvenience to smokers is no ex-
emption.
City of Tucson vs. Alfredo Montano —
Held by Judge Cowan that when one's mask is in the wash, it is no ex-
emption from wearing it. Also that a pink muffler is not a legal
substitute for a mask.[16]

Each of the defendants was fined ten dollars. A reporter noted that
all of them "fought hard for their ten spot, but the odds were against
them." S. Kogas, the Greek, was the only defendant who paid cheerful-
ly. He remarked that he was "glad to give a Christmas present to the
city." Despite the numerous arrests, the mask ordinance continued to
be disregarded. Many people preferred taking a chance that a
policeman would not appear, but "all have masks handy for an
emergency." Policemen often traveled in pairs to add to the weight of
testimony, and convictions mounted. The *Citizen* declared that "if the
order is kept in force long enough, the city overdraft will be paid and
Tucson will be out of the red."[17]

John Mets, prominent Tucson banker and civic leader, was arrested
on December 18. In fact, he was arrested so many times on that day
that he lost count. Mets insisted on ignoring the masking order, his
"visage not being decorated with even a wisp of gauze." And when it
became known that Mets wanted to make a test case of his citation for
not wearing an anti-influenza mask, he was hailed as a "champion" by
many of his fellow citizens. Mets, who had just returned from an extended eastern trip, vehemently disagreed with the Tucson health
authorities on the subject of masking. "To be plain," the *Citizen* noted,
he "regards it as a filthy practice." In an interview, Mets declared that
"masks are not being worn in any of the large cities of the east. I have
visited Chicago, New York, Washington and other large cities," and
"physicians are inserting half-page advertisements in the newspapers
advising their patients not to wear masks." In observing Tucson, Mets
had noticed many violators of the masking ordinance. "Look about this

bank," he said, as he surveyed the working force of the Arizona National and Merchants' Bank and Trust Company, "do you see anybody
who is obeying the law?" The *Citizen* reporter looked around, and
"saw that 90 percent were not. There were masks in plenty, but they
did not cover the nose or the mouth in many instances." Of course,
there were no policemen around. "I cannot do my work with one of
those things on," continued Mets. And that "gentleman over there, who
wears glasses, cannot keep his on, as his breath clouds up his lenses and
obscures his vision." The masking order, he concluded, "is impracticable in a dozen situations."

Found guilty by Judge Cowan, Mets appealed to superior court,
where his case was heard by Judge Samuel L. Pattee. Counsel for the
defense John H. Campbell stated that the city charter did not include a
provision for an emergency clause, thus the mask ordinance was illegal. Campbell also argued that since the ordinance was still being
advertised, it could not yet go into effect. Finally, he declared that the
ordinance was unconstitutional because it made an exception of school
children, who were not compelled to wear the masks in the school
rooms, thus it represented class legislation and should be declared invalid. Campbell also demurred on the ground that the requirement
was unreasonable. On December 21, Judge Pattee decided that the city
did have the right to pass an "emergency ordinance" for "immediate
enforcement." In cases of emergency, the court noted, the "specified
period of advertising is not necessary." Up to this point, Judge Pattee's
decision was regarded as a victory for supporters of the mask ordinance, but the issue of class legislation remained.

Defense counsel Campbell contended that the mask ordinance constituted class legislation in that it discriminated in favor of school
children by not requiring them to wear masks in the school rooms. City
attorney F. H. Bernard argued that the distinction made was one of environment and not of class. The sanitary conditions under which the
children study, he asserted, precluded the danger of infection which
existed in other public places. Campbell stated that the only presump-
tion he could draw from the ordinance was that "the germs would not
go near the public or private school buildings." Having "much fun at
the expense of the 'flubugs,'" the *Star* noted, defense lawyer Campbell
designated them "by the opprobrious term of 'low brow germs, not
desirous of a higher education.'" Judge Pattee ruled that the influenza
masking order was invalid. According to the court, the mask ordinance
represented class legislation, in that school children were exempted

from wearing masks. His ruling meant that flu masks were no longer compulsory in Tucson. Judge Pattee did not take up the question of whether the mask order was a reasonable one, for he "could not see how a person not a physician could reach a basis for determination." He admitted that some orders by a board of health, such as "wearing a gunny sack over the head or a suit of armor, would be patently unreasonable," but in the case of the flu mask he was wary of accepting the responsibility of determining its "reasonableness."

The city council or the board of health could go ahead and reestablish mask wearing by the simple process of including the schools under the term of a new ordinance or order. Meanwhile, the masks came off on December 24, the day before Christmas, and few Tucsonians protested. Even Judge Cowan must have been relieved. On December 21 he had been wearing his mask while riding on a streetcar, in accordance with the law, when he saw a boy riding a bicycle while holding on to the handrail of the streetcar for locomotion. As this was against a city ordinance, Judge Cowan moved to put his head out of a window and warn the boy. Unfortunately, his head crashed through the window pane; due to the fact that he did not see that the window was closed, because his glasses had become blurred from his breathing, by reason of the mask.

What course the city council or the board of health would now take regarding the epidemic in Tucson provoked discussion, but since the epidemic was slackening, most people did not foresee any further masking orders. A *Citizen* editorial, entitled "Good Riddance," thanked Judge Pattee for making "all hearts merry at the Christmas season by holding that the ordinance requiring every citizen to wear a rag over his nose and mouth is invalid." His "wisdom is apparent," and all should "compliment him in the name of humanity for his just decision." In Tucson, the paper declared, "the mask was never popular. Few had any faith in it." The ordinance "was incapable of enforcement. No matter how many citizens the city authorities might have taken to the lock-up, nor how many fines they imposed, they could never have brought about the general observance of masking." As "soon as the police were out of sight, the mask was dropped below the nose or down on the chin and not adjusted until danger approached." The city "copied the practice of masking from San Francisco. Some city health officers there sent a telegram telling what wonderful results San Francisco obtained from masking, and Tucson fell for it as it falls for every fad."

On Christmas day, the board of health warned of holiday crowds, and advised masking, but it also announced that no further action would be taken, pending developments. As Dr. Clyne put it, "there is no disposition at present on the part of the board to arbitrarily make use of its authority to press the issue by asking the city council to re-enact the mask ordinance in a constitutional form." By January 1, only two or three cases of Spanish influenza a day were being reported, and generally it was felt that the "flu menace" no longer existed in Tucson.[18]

At the same time, the disease was devastating Phoenix, the capital city of Arizona. As conditions worsened in Phoenix and improved in Tucson, leaders in the latter city began to suggest that the Arizona State Legislature hold its annual session in January 1919 in Tucson rather than in Phoenix. "Bring the legislature here," the *Star* declared on January 8, "if it decides to skip the 'Flu Haven' of Phoenix this month." Tucson "will be glad to have the legislature and to relieve the Phoenix people of the embarrassment as well as alarm they must feel in asking a body of prominent men, accompanied in not a few instances by their families, to assemble and live in a pest house." The "only argument against the proposal is that the luxury and convenience of Tucson and its accommodations might spoil the attendants to such an extent that we might find it difficult to keep them from establishing the capital here permanently, a course that none of us could view as just the right thing under the circumstances of the helplessness of Phoenix, upon her back, as it were, mortally stricken."

A day later, state legislators from Pima County and Tucson Chamber of Commerce officials issued a joint statement declaring that there existed "no disposition or intention to antagonize Phoenix or Maricopa County, and that the invitation to the legislature to hold its sessions in Tucson would not be extended unless the legislature decided not to meet in Phoenix." The statement pointed out that "although the idea was popular among the leading citizens of Tucson, that relations between Tucson and Phoenix have been consistently pleasant and cooperative for several years and that no fight should be made to secure the legislature for Tucson, notwithstanding the honor of entertaining the state's lawmakers and the material profit that would accrue from having so many visitors." The state legislature met in Phoenix on January 12, and by that date the influenza epidemic was waning in the capital city. A proposal in the legislature to recess until the disease disappeared received "scanty approval," and that select body of Arizonans continued to function in Phoenix. In Tucson, life had returned to normal. The Spanish influenza epidemic of 1918, a medical emergency and a trying experience, was over. As in many other cities, the influenza epidemic passed from Tucson as inexplicably as it had arrived.[19]

The impact of the Spanish influenza epidemic on Tucson was tremendous — as it had been in Albuquerque and El Paso. People in that southern Arizona city responded in a number of ways, some commendable, some not so commendable. The Tucson experience illustrates just how difficult it is to get everybody to join together in a common cause, however, worthy. Most citizens were cooperative, though, even if some did respond in a negative manner. Volunteer work in Tucson was as impressive as it was in other cities of the region and the nation. Phoenix residents, for example, commented favorably on the valuable aid rendered by volunteers in their sister city to the south. On the other hand, they were far less appreciative of the efforts of certain promoters to have the capital of Arizona moved to Tucson for "health reasons."

※　　　※　　　※

Chapter V

PHOENIX

Not Once But Twice

In September 1918, Phoenix was the leading city in Arizona, and the second largest in the Southwest. With a population approaching 28,000, the city served as the capitol as well as the commercial and industrial hub of the state. Located in the center of the rich, irrigated Salt River Valley, the most productive agricultural region in the Southwest, it was also recognized as a health haven and a winter tourist attraction. And as in other cities of the region at the time, the big news was World War I. Headlines such as "Americans and French Pushing Back Hun Forces" and "Americans and French Advance 7 Miles and Capture 12 Towns and 5,000 Prisoners" appeared regularly on the front pages of Phoenix newspapers. And local volunteers worked in liberty bond drives and for the Red Cross. Few people paid much attention to the occasional reports regarding the spread of Spanish influenza around the world.[1]

On September 29, Dr. Orville Harry Brown, state superintendent of public health, issued a warning about the disease, and suggested ways to avoid it. He emphasized the importance of enforcing city laws against spitting in public places. Every effort, he declared, should be made "to abolish this filthy and dangerous practice." Brown considered spitting "a common and widespread means of spreading influenza and other respiratory ailments," and he called upon "patriotic citizens" to aid the police by reporting violations.

On October 1, Dr. Brown urged that people refrain from kissing in Phoenix. This "sober and serious advice," noted the *Arizona Republican*, must be followed "while influenza is lurking about." It "makes no difference whether people are engaged to be married and have a perfect right to display affection in this manner." It "must not be indulged in, either upon the lips or the hand, unless they are willing to run the risk of contracting the Spanish influenza which is making serious headway throughout the country." Other preventative measures urged by Dr. Brown included the following: "Wash hands after shaking hands with another person. Don't startle that person by running right off to a washbowl, but get to one as soon as you can, when that person is not looking. Use your own drinking cup. Carry it with you. Wash the cup frequently. Sterilize your dishes. Keep clean in every way and keep everything about you clean. Be careful not to be in front of a person coughing or sneezing."[2]

Dr. Brown urged particular caution when coming into contact with coughers and sneezers. As he put it, "coughing and sneezing, except behind a handkerchief, is as great a sanitary offense as promiscuous spitting, and should be equally condemned." Although Brown and other Phoenix medical men expected the disease to hit the city, they hoped to prepare the public for its arrival. Strict sanitary precautions on the part of everyone, it was asserted, would "prevent the disease from spreading to any great extent." Institutions as well as individuals were encouraged to cooperate; for example, the State Board of Health adopted specific regulations to help secure sanitary conditions in public eating and drinking establishments. Owners of other businesses were asked to participate in the community effort. Theatre owners, for instance, could help by keeping their establishments "scrupulously clean." In theatres, Brown declared, attendants and patrons should be "on the lookout to see that no one spits on the floors, or sneezes promiscuously," and "every place touched by the hand of the public should be washed with hot water and soap after the performances." Brown concluded: "If prepared, there is no need for the people of this city to become unduly alarmed over the prospect of an epidemic of Spanish influenza."[3]

By October 5, Arizona was being invaded by the Spanish influenza, and there were at least twelve cases in Phoenix. The next day the Maricopa County Medical Society, upon the advice of Surgeon General Rupert Blue of the United States Public Health Service, recommended to city officials that all public and private schools, along with all churches, theatres, and other public meeting places be closed because of the "flu menace." It also urged that all public gatherings be indefinitely postponed. On October 7, the city commission passed an ordinance stating that "during the prevalence of any contagious, infectious, epidemic or endemic disease, all schools, theatres, moving picture shows, dance halls, pool halls, and other places of amusement shall be closed and no public meetings or assemblies of any kind shall be permitted to be held within the city." Any person found guilty of violating the provisions of the ordinance could be punished by a fine of not more than $300 or imprisonment not to exceed ninety days, or both fine and imprisonment. Drafted by city attorney Richard E. Sloan, the ordinance was initiated in response to the immediate community problem of Spanish influenza. It also was far-reaching in its scope and designed to be a permanent instrument to be used in the future if it became necessary to "safeguard the public against epidemic disease."

At the same time, the ordinance brought economic hardship to some citizens. At the city commission meeting, it was said that "at least 75 people will be thrown out of employment for an indefinite period by the closing of the theatres alone." Representatives of the theatres stated that they were not protesting, but they urged that the theatres be opened as soon as possible to save them from as much financial loss as possible. As a result of the ordinance, one observer declared, "the Columbia Theatre will lose at least $1,000 a week." The city commission sympathized with the theatre owners and other business interests, but most members went along with Dr. A. B. Nichols when he noted that it seemed "better to prevent now than to be sorry later."[4]

By October 10, Phoenix listed 100 cases of Spanish influenza, but health authorities remained hopeful that preventative measures would keep the epidemic from getting out of hand. "Conditions here are different than in other places where the disease has become a severe epidemic," stated Dr. Frederick T. Fahlen of the United States Public Health Service. Phoenix "has a warm climate, and even at this time of year the people sleep either outdoors or with all the windows open. This is favorable to only a light epidemic." To keep it a light epidemic, however, the people "must not lower their guard for a moment." All precautionary measures must be taken until "all danger has passed."

Fifteen people had died in Phoenix because of Spanish influenza by October 15. On that day, at least 150 cases of the disease existed in the city. "This is not a total by any means," declared the *Republican*, "as more than one-third of the city of Phoenix lies outside of the corporate limits where dwell the large part of the Mexican population among whom there are numerous cases of the disease." Many of the most serious cases were Mexicans, Dr. Fahlen pointed out, because the "crowded conditions in which the poorer class of Mexicans live and their low disease-resisting power on account of improper nourishment make them more susceptible to the disease than persons living under more favorable circumstances."⁵

The situation was bleak, and getting worse. Phoenix Union High School football games, and the State Fair, held each fall in Phoenix, were indefinitely postponed. With the number of Spanish influenza cases in Phoenix increasing, the need for medical personnel and facilities mounted. Unfortunately, six doctors and thirteen nurses had left the city to help meet the crisis in the more remote parts of Arizona. The *Republican* announced that "any person ill with influenza in need of assistance or care will receive prompt attention by notifying the Red Cross Influenza Committee." The committee, under the direction of John D. Loper, also determined to open an emergency hospital for flu victims, and on October 19, the Phoenix Women's Club offered the use of its building. The Sisters of Mercy also volunteered for use a new wing of St. Joseph's Hospital to supplement the emergency hospital being created in the Women's Club building. The wing, according to Dr. E. Payne Palmer, could "comfortably accommodate 50 cases and it is particularly adapted for treatment of the disease." Designed for "tubercular patients," the wing "has been built especially with a view of giving the patients fresh air and sunlight needed for the treatment of influenza."

A survey of the city, including the Mexican districts, found that many influenza cases remained "unattended and poverty stricken." Those who did not resist were taken to the Women's Club emergency hospital, where they were treated by Dr. Ancil Martin and his staff of volunteers. The Red Cross women of Phoenix, under the supervision of Mrs. Baron Goldwater, provided the hospital with a variety of goods, including clothing and bedding.⁶

The Women's Club emergency hospital soon became crowded. It even cared for prisoners from local jails who had contracted Spanish influenza. Not every patient appreciated the place. One of them, Pancho Marino, during his first evening in the hospital, lay near a patient who died during the night. A short time later another patient told him that two men had earlier died in the bed that he was occupying. When yet another man died near him, Marino became frightened and, clad only in a nightgown, leaped out of his bed and took off running. Guards, who mistakenly thought Marino was a hospitalized jail prisoner, fired several shots and chased him for two blocks before he disappeared into an alley. Three days later, Marino was found under some mesquite bushes at Seventh Avenue and Roosevelt Street. He was in "fairly good shape," according to police, despite the exposure. The police rushed him back to the emergency hospital where he received "proper attention."[7]

Despite the precaution, the epidemic in the Arizona capital kept spreading. On November 8, the *Republican* announced that so far 970 cases, with 54 deaths, had been reported within the Phoenix corporate limits. The day before, another single-day record had been set with 74 cases and four deaths reported. The hospitals were busier than ever, and two big tents, each with a capacity of twenty beds, were erected on the lot north of the Women's Club, as an annex to the emergency hospital. "The people of Phoenix are facing a crisis," declared the *Republican*. The Spanish influenza epidemic "has reached such serious proportions that it is the first problem before the people." The paper stated that "business houses are being compelled to close because there are not enough employees to do the work. Almost every home in the city has been stricken with the plague." The *Republican* called for more "fearless men and women to serve in the cause of humanity."[8]

All kinds of "treatments" were employed to help the afflicted. At one point, Dr. Orville Harry Brown commandeered some illegal whiskey from the county sheriff's office to use in fighting the epidemic. "We will not hesitate in using anything that will relieve suffering and bring the desired relief," declared the state superintendent of public health, and "if, after experiments, we are convinced that the medicinal properties of whiskey are a valuable agency in combatting the disease we will use it as a medicine whenever possible and whenever practical." On November 7, the *Arizona Gazette*, a Phoenix newspaper, noted the success of the experiments, and announced that "several hundred gallons of intoxicating beverages, seized by Sheriff W. H. Wilky and his deputies during the past two months, are now subject to consumption by the sufferers of this county by reason of a recent health order." The report continued: "One must be a legitimate sufferer before he can be taken into consideration at the dispensing bureau at the sheriff's office." Doctors "do not hesitate in issuing certificates for whiskey whenever they are in the belief that the individual can benefit from said treatment."

About $80,000 worth of whiskey seized in raids on bootleggers was stored in the sheriff's office. "If these intoxicating liquors will in any way give aid in suppressing the epidemic or will relieve suffering," Sheriff Wilky said, "I will not hesitate in issuing it upon presentation of a doctor's certificate." At the same time, the sheriff told the *Gazette* reporter that he "hadn't better write anything about that or we'll be so swamped with inquiries and demands that it will take a small army to maintain order at our office." On November 9, the *Republican* observed that the "sheriff's office for the past two days has been besieged with plain citizens, claiming to be almost dead from influenza, and by doctors, requesting whiskey for use in treatment of patients."[9]

Some of these patients, no doubt, participated in the big victory celebration on November 11. "Huns Sign Armistice, World War Is Over" read the headline in the *Republican*. A "parade a mile long rounded the streets of the city," a reporter wrote, while "church bells rang, guns were fired, and the people, who quickly filled the downtown streets, cheered and yelled and cheered again." There was also good news on the epidemic front. On November 14, the State Board of Health, after a meeting with city and county health officers, had adopted a plan to hasten the reopening of closed places in Arizona's cities. It stated that once seven conditions were met, and the number of Spanish influenza cases had sufficiently decreased, permission could be obtained from the Board to reopen the schools, churches, theatres, and other public gathering places. The seven conditions, published in local newspapers were:

1. There must be a universal, thorough cleaning of streets, alleys, yards and other places needing same.

2. A thorough scrubbing with hot water and soap or other approved method of cleaning, of all buildings, schools, churches, theatres, and other places where public meetings are held.

3. Placards for display must be printed and distributed to houses where influenza patients are located.

4. Conspicuous posters must be put prominently in all public places, calling attention to the dangers of coughing, sneezing, spitting, hand-shaking, and kissing, the use of dishes, glasses, and other tableware which have not been thoroughly washed in hot water since their previous use.

5. Inspection must be made by competent persons appointed by local health officers to ascertain if the food and drinking places are giving proper attention to the washing of their dishes and glasses, and other utensils used in preparation and serving of food and drink.

6. Receptacles must be placed upon the streets at such places and in such numbers as may be necessary to serve as sputum basins. A

prominent sign should be placed over each receptable, calling attention to the necessity of spitting in the receptacle and not upon the sidewalk or street or other inappropriate place.

7. An effort must be made to induce everybody to take the influenza vaccine. This effort must be honest, serious and systematic.[10]

The number of Spanish influenza cases in Phoenix continued to increase, and the city remained closed. Other Salt River Valley towns also experienced increases; their hospitals, like those in the capital city, were filled with patients, and all of them needed more doctors and nurses. At the same time, businessmen suffered financial losses and complained about the lack of success in the efforts to control the epidemic. Theatre owners, for example, stated that they were prepared to comply with all of the conditions of the plan, but they resented the provision that called for evidence of a decrease in influenza cases in Phoenix before places of business could be reopened. They declared it was a requirement over which they had no control. As George W. Barrows, a business spokesman put it, "apparently the influenza strikes where it chooses, regardless of precaution." He reminded health authorities that the Spanish influenza epidemic "had not lessened," but was "getting worse" despite the fact that the theatres had been closed for six weeks. Dr. Brown, speaking for most of the medical community, insisted that it was necessary to continue "all present precautionary methods to properly safeguard against a more serious epidemic of Spanish influenza." Not only were "proper sanitary methods, vaccinations and a partial quarantine" necessary, but he also suggested citizens be ordered to wear anti-germ masks. He read a telegram from Dr. William Hassler of San Francisco, in which the California health official stated that "by the use of influenza masks the number of new cases to be reported in that city had dropped from 2,000 to practically nothing in 20 days."[11]

The *Republican* announced a new two-day record of 303 cases on November 19, and it lamented that since October 10 there had been at least 1620 cases, with 88 deaths in Phoenix. The Associated Charities, a local voluntary organization, kept busy providing for the flu victims who were also indigent, but more help was needed. The *Gazette* called for more volunteers to respond to the "appeal which comes from hundreds of homes where one or more of the family are ill with the disease." It also urged all doctors to report cases immediately, noting that "only 50 percent of the prevalent cases in the city have been reported to authorities." At the same time, it commended Dr. A. B. Nichols, county health officer, for "taking steps to safeguard the outlying districts." Nichols had ordered "special deputies" to be stationed on all the main highways leading into the city. All traffic headed for Phoenix had to be halted, so as to determine which commuters had sufficient reason to enter the city. "If it is learned that the individual is merely coming to Phoenix to rest or visit, he will be turned back," disclosed Nichols, but "if he has actual business here, he will be permitted to continue his way." He told families from outside of Phoenix to stay home, and he promoted more mail-order business transactions.[12]

In the city, a citizens' committee was formed to "encourage" people to abide by the rules and regulations. Special police were ordered to "prevent the gathering of groups or crowds," and to "warn proprietors of business establishments to allow each customer at least 1,200 cubic feet of air space." Inspectors canvassing the city for influenza cases were told to place "quarantine cards" on each house containing a case. Victims not receiving attention at home were removed to emergency hospitals. In addition to cleaning up residential neighborhoods (some of which had not been touched for months), the streets, sidewalks and gutters of the downtown district were flushed with water in "an effort to drive the influenza germ out of Phoenix." A campaign was waged against those "who defy the city ordinance against spitting promiscuously on streets or sidewalks, in stores or anywhere except in spittoons and gutters."[13]

On November 25, the citizens' committee reported to a group of physicians, and all agreed that considerable progress had been made in combating the spread of influenza. Indeed, it was generally conceded that Phoenix was now a "cleaner city" than it had been for a long time. However, in order that even greater progress might be made, and so that the city could be opened again as soon as possible, it was decided to enact and enforce a mask order.

"Masks for everyone who appears in the streets of Phoenix," declared the *Republican*. "No one is to be exempted," stated the citizens' committee, and it went on to assert that "if the wearing of the influenza mask is of benefit to any single individual in this epidemic, it is good for all." At this time, there were 650 reported cases of influenza in the city, and it was felt by health authorities that a mask order was needed. The masks could be obtained at drug stores for ten cents or they could be easily made. The "principal thing," according to the citizens' committee, was that "each person, if he or she appears on the streets of the city, must have the lower portion of the face concealed, so that the transfer of influenza germs from one person to another by the means of coughing, sneezing or too close contact will be impossible." Two different kinds of masks met the approval of local physicians. One involved six thicknesses of gauze, 10 inches long and 8 inches wide. Pucker the ends, then knot a tape around each puckered end to be used in tying on the mask. The other suitable mask required a clean, close textured handkerchief, folded diagonally once from the corner, placed with the middle of the fold just below the eyes with the ends knotted at the back of the neck, and worn like "a highwayman's mask." All masks, of course, were to be kept fresh.

The citizens' committee reported that all doctors in the Phoenix area were "unanimous in favor of the universal wearing of the mask," and leading local citizens voiced their agreement. "San Francisco has adopted the influenza mask and is making headway against the influenza epidemic," stated Joe E. Rickard, who had just returned from a visit to the California city. "San Francisco has had a mighty bad time with the Spanish influenza," he said, and "it was getting worse and worse, and the city was in just about the condition Phoenix is now. They adopted the influenza mask, made everyone wear it in the streets and it has made a great difference. In a short time the number of new cases had fallen considerably."[14]

In spite of some criticism, the order of the city board of health went into operation on schedule. The notice of the regulation, issued November 26, declared that during the present epidemic of influenza, and until further orders, "no person shall frequent the streets, business houses or other public and semi-public places within the city of Phoenix, unless a gauze or cloth mask is worn over the nose and mouth in such a manner that the act of breathing is done through such a mask." The order was issued under the provisions of Arizona law that also called for the punishment of violators, including a fine not to exceed $100, or thirty days in jail, or both. "Individual homes are the only places left where a person may leave off his or her mask and escape punishment," noted the *Republican*. The ultimate purpose of the regulation, health authorities pointed out again and again, "was to wipe out the epidemic and make possible a general resumption of business." Considering the situation, they insisted that "the end more than justified the means."

"A city of masked faces," reported the *Republican* on November 27, "a city as grotesque as a masked carnival." The citizens' committee estimated that "95 percent of everyone who appeared on the streets were properly equipped with the influenza masks." At the same time, not every individual adhered to the order. Some "cautiously permitted their masks to dangle from one ear while they smoked." Other smokers cut holes in their masks to make room for their cigarettes, cigars, and pipes. Some diners, having trouble eating in restaurants with their masks on, discarded them. Also, every sort of mask could be seen on the streets. A few people used bailing wire to construct masks that resembled "muzzles" and one person put together a mask that looked like a "football nose guard." No mask, however, attracted as much attention as one seen on a woman on Washington Street. "Whether it was a tin can or a jelly glass hanging over her nose could not be ascertained," declared the *Gazette*, but "it was the size of a Happy Hooligan hat." The *Republican* reported: "'Flu germ' is the gauze mask worn by Miss Marion Grau, an office worker. He was noted on the lower left hand corner of the mask and he took the form of a little red devil." The paper announced that "the new fad among the merry maids of the mask is to conceive their own idea of the flu germ and embroider him on their masks." A touch of individualism helped to ease the tension in a city where friends of long standing often failed to recognize each other with their masks on. As one local "poet" put it:

> Owing to the cussed 'flu'
> If you want to know who's who,
> You will have to ask
> 'What is that behind the mask?'[15]

To make matters worse, the sheriff's office was running out of whiskey. The "epidemic has played havoc with the stock of contraband whiskey in the care of Sheriff W. H. Wilky," the *Gazette* announced on November 28, "or rather whiskey that was formerly under his care." Before the epidemic made its appearance in Phoenix, Sheriff Wilky had under his care "approximately 10,000 pints of confiscated liquors," but most of it "has already been consumed by sufferers of the disease." It was considered a very serious matter that the epidemic might outlast the supply of whiskey, and the sheriff was directed to prevent such a tragedy from occurring. Moreover, Phoenix experienced the quietist Thanksgiving Day in its history on November 28. There was little to attract the people from their homes. Thanksgiving church services were not allowed, but special Thanksgiving Day leaflets provided by the various churches were used in celebrations held in many homes. Comforting news appeared in the *Gazette* on November 30, when a report

showed 583 cases of influenza in Phoenix, a decrease of 16 from the
report of November 27.[16]

Because of favorable reports announcing fewer and fewer influenza
cases in the city, and acting on the recommendation of the Maricopa
County Medical Society, the board of health on December 3 cancelled
the mask order. At that time, there were 475 cases of the disease in
Phoenix, a decrease of 108 cases from the November 30 report. It also
was decided on December 8 to lift the ban on public gatherings, depen-
dent upon the continued improvement of influenza conditions in the
city. On December 4, the citizens' committee report listed 347 cases in
Phoenix, a decrease of 128 from the preceding day, and the "biggest
drop since the appearance of the epidemic." The future looked good.
"There can be no question that the reopening of business of all kinds in
the city will be generally welcomed." the *Gazette* declared, "A re-
juvenated Phoenix is ready to return to the activity that was inter-
rupted and to proceed with greater fervor in its own upbuilding and
furthering the prosperity of the Salt River Valley and the state."

"We are going to open and we are going to open with a bang," yelled
one theatre owner. "The people of Phoenix are hungry for amusement.
They have been deprived for many weeks. There has been little for
them to do except stay home. While there is no place like home, home
must have its contrasts and diversions to be appreciated."[17]

A few critics believed that Phoenix risked a "second wave" of influenza by acting prematurely. A county official hoped that "history will not
repeat and Phoenix suffer as other places have suffered by taking action
too soon." It had happened in Denver and San Francisco and other
cities in the United States "where the ban was lifted too early." On
December 8, the "starved pleasure-loving public" turned out in
Phoenix. Movies such as "Manhattan Madness" at the Columbia
Theatre, "Crashing Through To Berlin" at the American, and "Her
Price" at the Lamar, attracted capacity crowds. Church notices reap-
peared in the papers and clergymen reminded members of their congregations "to bring what you would have given these weeks and we
will recover from our financial loss much sooner." The *Republican*
noted that Phoenix "society" was beginning to enjoy "the most brilliant
events in the social history of the city." The "winter tourist season is getting into full-swing now, and hotels are filling up," observed the
Gazette on December 12. "At the Adams Hotel yesterday, guests from
13 states were registered, a large proportion of them coming from the
east. Other hotels of the city had similar experiences."[18]

People danced and club members met, but the schools did not reopen. Due to the reopening of the theatres and other places of business, the school board decided to keep the schools closed until December 30. "We would rather wait a little longer," a spokesman for the board declared, "than to reopen the schools and then be compelled to close them again, as has been done in Los Angeles, San Diego and several other places." In the meantime, 600 Phoenix Union High School students continued to take correspondence lessons; indeed, the program served as a model for high schools throughout the nation.[19]

On December 14, only 160 influenza cases were reported in Phoenix, and jubilant health authorities announced that the predicted "second wave" of the disease had been averted. It "is the consensus of opinion," stated Dr. H. K. Beauchamp, city health officer, "that the anticipated revival of the epidemic attendant upon the reopening of the theatres, churches, etc., has been effectually prevented through the measures adopted to combat the dreaded invasion." This belief "is based upon the fact that in practically every instance recorded the recurrence has succeeded the first abatement of the influenza within three to five days. Not only are the signs of a new 'peak' lacking, but the indications are that a few days more will see the complete annihilation of the plague." During the week before Christmas, the streets and stores of Phoenix had filled with holiday shoppers, but on December 28, the *Republican* announced a total of 102 influenza cases in the city, and remarked that the number of cases declined despite the large Christmas season crowds. The school board, noting the figures, decided to go ahead as planned and open the schools on December 30. "Every classroom has been carefully cleaned and fumigated," stressed superintendent of public schools John D. Loper, and "during school hours nurses will be in each room watching the pupils for signs of illness."[20]

The first unfavorable report came on December 29, with 115 cases, 13 more than the preceding day. On January 1, 1919, the *Gazette* announced that the "second wave" of the epidemic had hit Phoenix, with 216 influenza cases in the city. Hoping to "profit from experience," the board of health and the city commission imposed restrictive measures on the community that were practically identical to those enforced during the first wave of the epidemic. Once again, the authorities prohibited public and private gatherings, the schools closed, and an absolute quarantine was placed on all houses containing influenza cases. Masks had to be worn by all persons coming in contact with the disease. Fifty special policemen received instructions to help regular officers enforce the rules and regulations. January 8 "found Phoenix completely in the grip of its second influenza epidemic, with a second strict quarantine and the city virtually closed up," reported the *Republican*. On that day, the total number of influenza cases in the city reached 550, a jump of 450 in ten days. The old record of 634, set in October during the first wave, was broken two days later when the *Republican* announced a total of 712 cases in the capital city.[21]

Some individuals and groups objected to the new rules and regulations. The theatre owners of Phoenix decided to test the validity of the new city ordinance that ordered the closing of their places of business. The doors of the Strand and Columbia theatres opened on January 8 and the owners were arrested. They were found guilty and fined, but they appealed to Superior Court, calling the case against them discriminatory. "If all places of business in the city were obliged to close," declared a statement by theatre owners, "we would gladly comply with the order to assist authorities in more quickly stamping out the disease." The theatre owners felt that they should not be "singled out from the many and made to pay, with our dollars and cents, that which we are not more responsible for than the others."

The *Gazette*, speaking for many residents of Phoenix, approved the strict quarantine of houses containing flu cases, but it also criticized the closing of places of amusement, notably the theatres. It stated that in New York and Chicago nothing was closed, but an absolute quarantine was established in each city. Phoenix, it declared, should follow the example of those two great cities, rather than "instilling fear into the hearts of every man, woman and child in the city by closing theatres and other meeting places."

At the same time, the total number of influenza cases in the city exceeded the high point of the first wave, and the hospitals were filled to capacity. The "need of another hospital to assist in the care of sufferers is becoming more and more apparent as each day passes," declared the *Republican*. The Women's Club emergency hospital experience and that of St. Joseph's had encouraged many residents to call for better health facilities in Phoenix; for example, a campaign was initiated to raise $100,000 to expand Arizona Deaconess Hospital in the city.

On January 11, the city ordinance providing for the closing of theatres and other places of public amusement was held to be unconstitutional by Judge R. C. Stanford. As he put it, "the law is discriminatory in that it singles out one business from another and infers that business is more responsible for the spread of influenza than any other form of business." In his opinion, there had been "great discrimination in this matter, and it is a well established principle of law that discriminatory legislation is unconstitutional." The decision removed closing regulations on theatres and other places of public gathering, but a strict quarantine on houses continued in force, and the schools did not reopen.[22]

On January 14, the daily influenza count showed for the first time during the second wave a decrease in cases, down from 714 to 639. With the favorable report, health officials expressed the opinion that the "crest of the flu wave has passed." Six days later, the *Gazette* reported 327 cases of the disease in Phoenix, and declared that the second attack of Spanish influenza seemed to be subsiding as rapidly as it had risen. By January 24, the day the schools reopened, the epidemic had reached a point where it was generally regarded as "a thing of the past." Quarantine regulations on individual cases remained, but the city seemed to be getting back to normal. By February 1, the count was down to 79, and on February 15, in response to an inquiry from New York, the *Republican* announced that it wanted "the world to know that Phoenix is now entirely free from influenza."[23]

The Spanish influenza epidemic hit El Paso harder than any other major urban center in the region, but Phoenix was the only one hit twice. Citizens of the Arizona capital were still celebrating the end of the first wave of the epidemic when a second wave sturck. The first wave produced a considerable number of volunteers, but during the second there was less willingness to serve. Cooperation between the public and private sectors declined. Critics, led by business interests who were losing money, challenged the effectiveness of the rules and regulations imposed upon the public and were successful in getting some of them removed by court action. At the same time, many local leaders realized the need to expand health-care facilities in Phoenix, and they continued to promote the development of those institutions in the city in order to provide better protection against future medical emergencies.

꙳   ꙳   ꙳

SUMMARY

The Spanish influenza epidemic entered the Southwest in force in October 1918, and its impact on the region and its towns and cities was considerable. The epidemic has been given little attention in the historiography of the Southwest because of the significance of World War I, but its importance to the social history of the region should not be overlooked. At the time, for many in the Southwest, as elsewhere in the nation, the most vicious enemy was the germ, not the German. The epidemic affected individuals and institutions on the local level in many ways; it brought out the best and the worst characteristics of the people and places involved.

In the cities of the Southwest, local leaders and local populations remained apathetic about the Spanish influenza epidemic until it hit home, but once it arrived they moved into action. Once the theory that the epidemic could not occur in the "health centers" of the "sunny Southwest" had proved to be incorrect, each community responded. Once aware that the disease had actually invaded their respective cities, local officials in the region tried every technique, procedure, and remedy that had been used elsewhere in the country to cure or slow the advance of the disease. All kinds of information, on how to avoid or survive influenza, was disseminated to the public and the press in the urban Southwest. Public gatherings were prohibited. All schools, churches, and places of public amusement were closed. Many citizens were inoculated with useless vaccines. (It was not until 1943 that the first successful vaccine against the flu was developed.) In Tucson and Phoenix, as in Denver, San Francisco, and other urban centers, city officials spent much time and effort trying to persuade people to wear anti-influenza masks. In the Arizona cities, local officials made the wearing of masks obligatory in all public places. With the public interest in mind, city officials such as Charles Davis of El Paso, Moise Bergman of Albuquerque, Meade Clyne of Tucson, and John D. Loper

[58]

of Phoenix fought the "Battle of the Flu." So did the editors of the *Morning Times* and the *Herald* in El Paso, the *Morning Journal* and the *Evening Herald* in Albuquerque, the *Star* and the *Citizen* in Tucson, and the *Republican* and the *Gazette* in Phoenix.

The great majority of urban Southwesterners appreciated the positive action utilized by local authorities to prevent the epidemic from spreading. Most obeyed the rules and regulations; many of those who did not were arrested and fined. Encouraged by the local press, the public for the most part cooperated, but as the epidemic continued, it affected commerce, industry, education, recreation, cultural events, religious services, elections, the war effort, and all other parts of the community. Local critics challenged the effectiveness of closing businesses, the use of masks, and other restrictions. The critics included businessmen and some newspaper editors who worried about the impact that the rules and regulations were having and would continue to have on the social, political, cultural, and economic life of the four cities. In some instances, notably in Tucson and Phoenix, enough pressure was brought to bear on officials by the press and the public to bring a halt to such restrictive measures as closing and masking orders. And in the end, the disease eventually slackened and then disappeared from all four cities for no known reason.

As in other cities around the nation, the war against the Spanish influenza was lost in the urban Southwest, but the battle was fought despite the lack of means to win. In test cases, the courts recognized the rights of the cities to issue emergency ordinances and to suspend ordinary procedures during crisis times such as lethal epidemics. Also, many urban Southwesterners gave of themselves in attempting to prevent the epidemic from spreading. Doctors and nurses, risking their own health, were overworked, but they learned from the experience. Community-minded volunteers contributed their services to victims of the disease throughout the ordeal, and received the satisfaction of lending a helping hand to the less fortunate fellow citizens in their hour of need. The able women of the urban Southwest, such as A. Louise Dietrich of El Paso, Sister Alma Louise Vogt of Albuquerque, Anna Blount of Tucson, and Mrs. Baron Goldwater of Phoenix, displayed a remarkable effort. Indeed, the soup kitchens and the emergency hospitals, however efficiently organized and coordinated, would have been of little use if the citizens had not volunteered their services. Individually and collectively they contributed food, clothing, and care to the victims of the epidemic. They played a large role in the development of such beneficial institutions as the Aoy School emergency hospital in El Paso and the Women's Club emergency hospital in Phoenix.

It became apparent to many of those involved in the crisis that the cities of the Southwest needed more public health professionals and public health facilities if they were to be adequately prepared to deal with medical emergencies in the future. The epidemic was a trying experience for the medical profession, and it pointed out the need for more scientific research and public education. As for the future, medical progress was forthcoming, but the social history of the Spanish influenza epidemic of 1918-1919 was soon forgotten. In the cities of the Southwest, as in other urban centers of the nation, most people preferred to remember World War I and victory, rather than the days of disease and defeat.

ఆ   ఆ   ఆ

NOTES

Chapter I — A NATIONAL DISASTER

1. The best account of the Spanish influenza epidemic experience on the international and national level is Alfred W. Crosby, Jr., *Epidemic and Peace, 1918* (Westport, Conn.: Greenwood Press, 1976). See also A. A. Hoehling, *The Great Epidemic* (Boston: Little, Brown & Co., 1961); William R. Noyes, "Influenza Epidemic, 1918-1919: A Misplaced Chapter in U.S. Social and Institutional History" (Ph.D. disst., University of California at Los Angeles, 1968); Joseph E. Persico, "The Great Spanish Flu Epidemic of 1918," *American Heritage* 27 (June 1976), 28-31, 80-85; Dorothy Ann Pettit, "A Cruel Wind: America Experiences the Pandemic Influenza, 1918-20" (Ph.D. disst., University of New Hampshire, 1976).
2. Crosby, *Epidemic and Peace*, pp. 6-7, 46-49, 74; Hoehling, *Great Epidemic*, pp. 30-32.
3. Hoehling, *Great Epidemic*, pp. 60-62, 75-78, 115-116; Crosby, *Epidemic and Peace*, pp. 48-49, 73-74, 80-85; Persico, "Epidemic of 1918," *American Heritage*, pp. 30-31, 80-83.
4. Edward Robb Ellis, *Echos of Distant Thunder: Life in the United States, 1914-1918* (New York: Coward, McCann & Geoghegan, Inc., 1975), pp. 466-467; Crosby, *Epidemic and Peace*, pp. 74-76; Pettit, "A Cruel Wind," pp. 115-125, 211-212.
5. Crosby, *Epidemic and Peace*, pp. 74-84, 96-97, 114-116; Hoehling, *Great Epidemic*, pp. 93-98; Noyes, "Influenza Epidemic," pp. 112-124.
6. Ellis, *Life in the United States*, pp. 463-464; Irwin Ross, "The Great Plague of 1918," *American History Illustrated* 3 (July 1968), p. 13; Hoehling, *Great Epidemic*, pp. 33-34, 72.

7. Hoehling, *Great Epidemic*, pp. 75-77; Ellis, *Life in the United States*, pp. 466-467; Crosby, *Epidemic and Peace*, pp. 84-85; Pettit, "A Cruel Wind," pp. 137-142.

8. Crosby, *Epidemic and Peace*, pp. 84-85, 106, 114; Pettit, "A Cruel Wind," pp. 269-270.

9. Noyes, "Influenza Epidemic," pp. 47-48, 257; Crosby, *Epidemic and Peace*, pp. 91-116, 323-325. See also Alfred W. Crosby, Jr., "The Pandemic of 1918," in June E. Osborn, ed., *Influenza in America, 1918-1976* (New York: Prodist, 1977), pp. 5-13.

10. The few studies concerned with the Spanish influenza epidemic experience on the international and national level do not discuss the Southwest. The regional and state survey histories of the area also do not discuss the epidemic. Moreover, as noted in the following chapters, the urban biographies of the four cities pay little or no attention to the epidemic.

Chapter II — EL PASO

1. The most comprehensive biography of El Paso, C. L. Sonnichsen, *Pass of the North: Four Centuries on the Rio Grande*, 2 vols. (El Paso: Texas Western Press of The University of Texas at El Paso, 1980), does not mention the Spanish influenza epidemic. Mario T. Garcia gives it one paragraph in his *Desert Immigrants: The Mexicans of El Paso, 1880-1920* (New Haven: Yale University Press, 1981). Both books provide valuable background material on the history of El Paso during World War I. See also Bradford Luckingham, *The Urban Southwest: A Profile History Of Albuquerque, El Paso, Phoenix, and Tucson* (El Paso: Texas Western Press, 1982), Chapter 3.

2. *El Paso Morning Times*, September 21, 24, 25, 28, October 4, 6, 1918; *El Paso Herald*, September 27, October 3, 4, 5, 7, 1918.

3. *El Paso Morning Times*, October 8, 9, 14, 1918; *El Paso Herald*, October 8, 9, 11, 12, 14, 1918; E. B. Rogers, M.D., "The Influenza Epidemic," *Southwestern Medicine* 2 (November, 1918), p. 7.

4. *El Paso Morning Times*, October 15, 17, 1918; *El Paso Herald*, October 15, 16, 1918.

5. *El Paso Morning Times*, October 16, 1918; *El Paso Herald*, October 16, 17, 1918; Garcia, *Desert Immigrants*. passim; Luckingham, *The Urban Southwest*, Chapter 3.

6. *El Paso Herald*, May 25, 1914; Oscar J. Martinez, *Border Boom Town: Ciudad Juarez since 1848* (Austin: University of Texas Press, 1978), Chapter 3; Garcia *Desert Immigrants*, Chapter 7; Luckingham, *The Urban Southwest*, Chapter 3.
7. *Ibid;* Garcia, *Desert Immigrants*, Chapter 7; Department of Planning, City of El Paso, *A Short History of South El Paso* (El Paso: Department of Planning, 1966), 15-21.
8. *El Paso Morning Times*, October 16, 17, 1918; *El Paso Herald*, October 16, 17, 1918. For a brief history of Aoy School, see Bertha A. Schaer, "An Historical Sketch of Aoy School" (Unpublished paper, The University of Texas at El Paso Library, 1951).
9. *El Paso Morning Times*, October 19, 1918; *El Paso Herald*, October 19, 1918.
10. *El Paso Morning Times*, October 19, 1918; *El Paso Herald*, October 16, 19, 1918. The Women's Charity Association of El Paso reorganized in 1915 to become the Associated Charities. Eddie Lou Miller, "The History of Private Welfare Agencies in El Paso, 1886-1930," (M.A. thesis: The University of Texas at El Paso, 1969), p. 67.
11. *El Paso Herald*, October 22, 23, 24, 1918; *El Paso Morning Times*, October 22, 23, 1918.
12. *El Paso Herald*, October 23, 24, 1918; *El Paso Morning Times*, October 23, 1918; Rogers, "Influenza Epidemic," *Southwestern Medicine*, p. 10.
13. *El Paso Morning Times*, October 23, 1918; *El Paso Herald*, October 23, 1918. See also Garcia, *Desert Immigrants*, p. 146.
14. *El Paso Morning Times*, October 27, 28, 29, 1918; *El Paso Herald*, October 25, 26, 28, 1918; R.L. Ramey, M.D., "The Surgical Side of the Flu," *Southwestern Medicine* 3 (October 1919), pp. 4-5.
15. *El Paso Morning Times*, October 29, 1918; *El Paso Herald*, November 1, 1918.
16. *El Paso Herald*, November 2, 1918; *El Paso Morning Times*, November 5, 1918.
17. *El Paso Herald*, November 5, 6, 15, 1918.
18. *El Paso Morning Times*, November 6, 1918; *El Paso Herald*, November 5, 1, 7, 1918. For a brief overview of welfare agencies in El Paso, see Helen Rainey, "A History of Organized Welfare in El Paso, 1892-1948," (M.A. thesis: The University of Texas at El Paso, 1949).

19. *El Paso Morning Times,* November 6, 1918; *El Paso Herald,* November 7, 1918.
20. *El Paso Morning Times,* November 9, 10, 11, 12, 1918; *El Paso Herald,* November 9, 11, 1918.
21. *El Paso Morning Times,* November 18, 19, 24, 1918; *El Paso Herald,* November 25, 29, 1918.
22. *El Paso Herald,* December 7, 10, 24, 1918, January 23, February 10, 1919; *El Paso Morning Times,* December 10, 20, 1918, January 31, 1919.

Chapter 3 — ALBUQUERQUE

1. The most comprehensive biography of Albuquerque, Marc Simmons, *Albuquerque: A Narrative History* (Albuquerque: University of New Mexico Press, 1982), includes one sentence on the epidemic, but it does provide some background material on the history of the city during World War I. See also Bradford Luckingham, *The Urban Southwest: A Profile History of Albuquerque, El Paso, Phoenix, and Tucson* (El Paso: Texas Western Press, 1982), Chapter 3. For a discussion of the epidemic in the state of New Mexico, see Richard Melzer, "A Dark and Terrible Moment: The Spanish Flu Epidemic of 1918 in New Mexico," *New Mexico Historical Review* 57 (July 1982), pp. 213-236.
2. *Albuquerque Morning Journal,* September 29, October 1, 1918.
3. (Albuquerque) *Evening Herald,* October 5, 1918; *Albuquerque Morning Journal,* October 5, 6, 1918.
4. *Evening Herald,* October 7, 8, 1918; *Albuquerque Morning Journal,* October 7, 8, 1918; Melzer, "New Mexico," *New Mexico Historical Review,* p. 215-216.
5. *Albuquerque Morning Journal,* October 13, 14, 1918; *Evening Herald,* October 16, 1918.
6. *Albuquerque Morning Journal,* October 17, 1918; *Evening Herald,* October 19, 1918; W.G. Hope, M.D., "Some Features of Influenza," *Southwestern Medicine* 4 (August 1920), p. 1-2.
7. *Albuquerque Morning Journal,* October 16, 17, 19, 20, 1918.
8. *Albuquerque Morning Journal,* October 19, 22, 24, 1918; *Evening Herald,* October 19, 1918.
9. *Albuquerque Morning Journal,* October 24, 25, 1918; *Evening Herald,* October 28, 1918; S.L. Burton, M.D., "The Prevention

of Influenza and Its Complications," *Southwestern Medicine* 3 (February 1919), p. 11.

10. *Albuquerque Morning Journal*, October 30, 31, November 3, 1918; *Evening Herald*, October 29, November 2, 1918.

11. *Evening Herald*, November 2, 6, 1918; *Albuquerque Morning Journal*, October 31, November 3, 1918.

12. *Evening Herald*, November 11, 12, 1918; *Albuquerque Morning Journal*, November 12, 15, 17, 1918.

13. *Albuquerque Morning Journal*, November 15, 1918.

14. *Albuquerque Morning Journal*, November 16, 17, 20, 24, 1918; Hope, "Influenza," *Southwestern Medicine*, pp. 1-2.

15. *Albuquerque Morning Journal*, November 17, 20, 24, 25, 26, 1918; *Evening Herald*, November 23, 1918; Melzer, "New Mexico," *New Mexico Historical Review*, p. 224.

16. *Albuquerque Morning Journal*, November 26, 27, 1918.

17. *Evening Herald*, November 28, December 3, 1918; *Albuquerque Morning Journal*, November 28, 30, December 2, 1918.

18. *Albuquerque Morning Journal*, December 4, 5, 6, 7, 13, 17, 1918; *Evening Herald*, December 7, 16, 18, 1918.

19. *Albuquerque Morning Journal*, November 30, December 12, 1918; *Evening Herald*, December 18, 1918; Melzer, "New Mexico," *New Mexico Historical Review*, pp. 229-232.

20. *Evening Herald*, January 8, 15, March 14, 1919; *Albuquerque Morning Journal*, January 10, 1919; *Laws of the State of New Mexico Passed by the Fourth Regular Session of the Legislature of the State of New Mexico, 1919* (Albuquerque: Albright & Anderson, 1919), Chapter 85, pp. 161-171.

21. *Albuquerque Morning Journal*, December 22, 1918, January 16, 19, 24, 1919; *Evening Herald*, February 10, 1919.

Chapter 4 — TUCSON

1. The two most comprehensive biographies of Tucson, C.L. Sonnichsen, *Tucson: The Life and Times of an American City* (Norman, Okla: University of Oklahoma Press, 1982), and John Bret Harte, *Tucson: Portrait of a Desert Pueblo* (Woodland Hills, Calif.: Windsor Publications, 1980), discuss the period of World War I in Tucson history, but Bret Harte does not mention the epidemic and Sonnichsen gives it one short paragraph. For the

World War I era, see also Bradford Luckingham, *The Urban Southwest: A Profile History of Albuquerque, El Paso, Phoenix and Tucson* (El Paso: Texas Western Press, The University of Texas, El Paso, 1982), Chapter 3.

2. (Tucson) *Arizona Daily Star*, October 5, 1918; *Tucson Citizen*, October 5, 1918.

3. *Arizona Daily Star*, October 10, 11, 1918; O.H. Brown, M.D., *Report of the Arizona State Board of Health For the Biennium January 1, 1917 to December 31, 1918* (Phoenix: Manufacturing Stationers, Inc., 1918), pp. 9-10.

4. *Arizona Daily Star*, October 11, 15, 1918; *Tucson Citizen*, October 10, 11, 22, 1918; Rupert Blue, "Spanish Influenza," *United States Public Health Service Supplement No. 34 to Public Health Reports September 28, 1918* (Washington: Government Printing Office, 1918).

5. *Arizona Daily Star*, October 17, 1918; *Tucson Citizen*, October 24, 1918.

6. *Tucson Citizen*, October 24, November 12, 1918; *Arizona Daily Star*, November 12, 1918.

7. *Arizona Daily Star*, November 16, 1918; "The Influenza Epidemic," *Bulletin Arizona Board of Health* 7 (April 1919), pp. 5-6.

8. *Arizona Daily Star*, November 16, 1918.

9. *Arizona Daily Star*, November 17, 1918; *Tucson Citizen*, November 17, 1918.

10. *Tucson Citizen*, November 19, 1918; *Arizona Daily Star*, November 19, 1918.

11. *Tucson Citizen*, November 20, 21, 22, 1918; *Arizona Daily Star*, November 22, 1918; Brown, *Report of the Arizona State Board of Health, 1917-1918*, pp. 10-11.

12. *Arizona Daily Star*, November 22, 23, 1918; *Tucson Citizen*, November 23, 1918.

13. *Tucson Citizen*, November 22, 25, 28, 30, 1918; *Arizona Daily Star*, November 29, 1918; "The Influenza Epidemic," *Bulletin Arizona Board of Health*, p. 16.

14. *Tucson Citizen*, December 1, 3, 1918; *Arizona Daily Star*, December 1, 3, 1918.

15. *Tucson Citizen*, December 4, 13, 14, 1918; *Arizona Daily Star*, December 4, 12, 13, 1918; W.W. Watkins, M.D., "The Influenza

Epidemic in Arizona," *Southwestern Medicine* 2 (November 1918), pp. 16-17.

16. *Arizona Daily Star*, December 17, 1918; *Tucson Citizen*, December 18, 1918; *Public Health Laws of the State of Arizona , 1916-1929* (Phoenix: State Board of Health, 1929), pp. 8-13.

17. *Tucson Citizen*, December 18, 19, 1918.

18. *Arizona Daily Star*, December 18, 20, 22, 24, 26, 1918; *Tucson Citizen*, December 19, 20, 22, 25, 1918, January 1, 1919.

19. *Arizona Daily Star*, January 8, 9, 12, 1919.

Chapter 5 — PHOENIX

1. G. Wesley Johnson, Jr., *Phoenix: Valley of the Sun* (Tulsa: Continental Heritage Press, 1982), devotes only one paragraph to the Spanish influenza epidemic, but it includes valuable material on the World War I period in the Arizona capital. See also Luckingham, *The Urban Southwest: A Profile History of Albuquerque, El Paso, Phoenix and Tucson* (El Paso: Texas Western Press, The University of Texas, El Paso, 1982), Chapter 3.

2. (Phoenix) *Arizona Republican*, September 29, 1918; "The Influenza Epidemic," *Bulletin of the Arizona State Board of Health* 7 (April 1919), pp. 5-6.

3. *Arizona Republican*, October 1, 3, 5, 1918; (Phoenix) *Arizona Gazette*, October 5, 1918.

4. *Arizona Republican*, October 5, 8, 1918; *Arizona Gazette*, October 7, 1918; Watkins, "The Influenza Epidemic in Arizona," *Southwestern Medicine* 2 (November 1918), pp. 16-17.

5. *Arizona Gazette*, October 10, 15, 1918; *Arizona Republican*, October 10, 15, 1918.

6. *Arizona Republican*, October 16, 17, 18, 19, 20, 22, 1918; *Arizona Gazette*, October 19, 22, 1918; O.H. Brown, M.D., *Report of the Arizona State Board of Health for the Biennium January 1, 1917, to December 31, 1918* (Phoenix: The Manufacturing Stationers, Inc., 1918), pp. 10-11.

7. *Arizona Republican*, November 3, 4, 6, 1918.

8. *Arizona Republican*, November 8, 1918.

9. *Arizona Gazette*, November 7, 9, 1918; *Arizona Republican*, November 8, 9, 1918.

10. *Arizona Gazette*, November 11, 1918; *Arizona Republican*, November 10, 11, 12, 1918.

11. *Arizona Republican*, November 12, 14, 1918; *Arizona Gazette*, November 13, 1918 Brown, *Report of the Arizona State Board of Health 1917-1918*, pp. 9-10.

12. *Arizona Republican*, November 19, 1918; *Arizona Gazette*, November 19, 1918.

13. *Arizona Gazette*, November 19, 20, 1918; *Arizona Republican*, November 20, 22, 23, 24, 1918.

14. *Arizona Republican*, November 26, 27, 28, 29, December 1, 1919; *Arizona Gazette*, November 27, 1918.

15. *Arizona Republican*, November 26, 27, 28, 29, December 1, 1918; *Arizona Gazette*, November 28, 1918; E.B. Rogers, M.D., "The Influenza Epidemic," *Southwestern Medicine* 2 (November 1918), p. 10.

16. *Arizona Gazette*, November 27, 30, 1918.

17. *Arizona Gazette*, December 3, 4, 5, 1918; *Arizona Republican*, December 3, 5, 1918.

18. *Arizona Republican*, December 6, 8, 9, 10, 12, 1918; *Arizona Gazette*, December 12, 16, 1918; W.W. Watkins, "Influenza Epidemic in Arizona," *Southwestern Medicine* 2 (November 1918), p. 17.

19. *Arizona Republican*, November 12, December 13, 15, 1918; *Arizona Gazette*. December 13, 1918.

20. *Arizona Republican*, December 14, 24, 27, 28, 1918; *Arizona Gazette*, December 16, 21, 26, 1918.

21. *Arizona Republican*, December 29, 1918; January 3, 4, 6, 7, 8, 10, 1919; *Arizona Gazette*, December 30, 1918, January 3, 6, 7, 8, 1919; George E. Goodrich, M.D., *State of Arizona, State Board of Health, Bienniel Report of the State Superintendent of Public Health, 1919-1920* (Phoenix: The Manufacturing Stationers, Inc., 1920), pp. 5-8.

22. *Arizona Republican*, January 8, 9, 10, 12, 1918; *Arizona Gazette*, January 7, 8, 11, 1918; "The Influenza Epidemic," *Bulletin Arizona Board of Health* 7 (April 1919), p. 16.

23. *Arizona Republican*, January 14, 16, 19, 22, 24, 27, February 1, 15, 1919; *Arizona Gazette*, January 16, 25, 1919.